I0440755

THE TRUTH ABOUT LIVING WITH

G6PD DEFICIENCY

ALSO BY DALE R. BAKER:

STAYING HEALTHY WITH G6PD DEFICIENCY:
A valuable reference guide for eating safely

Creator and web-master of
G6PDDEFICIENCY.ORG

THE TRUTH ABOUT LIVING WITH

G6PD DEFICIENCY

DALE R. BAKER

G6PD Publishing

Copyright © 2013 by Dale R. Baker

First Edition

All rights reserved. No part of this publication may be reproduced, distributed, or transmitted in any form or by any means, including photocopying, recording, or other electronic or mechanical methods, without the prior written permission of the publisher, except in the case of brief quotations embodied in critical reviews and certain other noncommercial uses permitted by copyright law. For permission requests, write to the publisher, addressed "Attention: Permissions Coordinator," at the address below.

Dale. R. Baker Publishing
P. O. Box 1167, San Andreas, CA 95249
Website: g6pddeficiency.org

Ordering Information: Quantity sales. Special discounts are available on quantity purchases by corporations, associations, and others. For details, contact the publisher at the address above.

Orders by U.S. trade bookstores and wholesalers. Please contact Dale R. Baker: Tel: (209) 662-0880 or visit g6pddeficiency.org

Printed in the United States of America

Publisher's Cataloging-in-Publication data

Baker, Dale R.

The Truth About Living with G6PD Deficiency : What Doctor's Don't Know / Dale R. Baker ; p. 88 cm.

ISBN-13: 978-1483999951
ISBN-10: 1483999955

1. G6PD Deficiency. 2. Health (genetic disorders). 3. Hemolytic Anemia 3. Favism 4. CNSHA.

14 13 12 11 10 / 10 9 8 7 6 5 4 3 2 1

DEDICATION

For my mother... because without her insight, her love and wisdom
I would not be here today.

Health is a birthright. Get involved. Claim it.

-Dr. Dorothy Ugundu, MD

Contents

PREFACE

In 2007 I started learning about G6PDD in earnest due to health problems I was experiencing and the medical profession's inability to tell me why, or even what was causing them. Although I thought I knew enough about G6PDD, I soon found out just how little I knew and how much damage ignorance had caused me.

Being a retired computer programmer, I naturally turned to my former profession for a way to tell others what I was learning and to learn from their experiences. Therefore, I started g6pddeficiency.org. Over the past six years, it has grown beyond anything I ever dreamed.

There have been thousands of people who have contributed to the website and the community's knowledge of G6PDD. This book is the result of their input, and our combined research and experiences. It explains what G6PDD is; why so few people know about it; how to be healthy; how you got it; how to keep from having reactions; how to protect your baby from complications; and many other things necessary to live a healthy life. There is much more to learn, and, expectantly, we will get the medical profession behind us at some point.

Over the years, I have heard many stories from people about their experience with G6PDD. Many ended in the tragic and unnecessary death of a loved one. Others left a child with permanent brain damage. Each of these stories has made me more determined to stop this tragic loss or impairment of human life. This book is written in their memory. May there never be another needless tragedy.

-Dale R. Baker

ACKNOWLEDGMENTS

I would like to thank the following people for their help
in writing this book:

Dr. Dorothy Ogundu.
She has been an inspiration and guide to me in my discovery of
the truth. To her goes my undying gratitude.

The thousands of people who have participated in the forum and
by email. Each of them has contributed to the world's knowledge
about G6PDD. Many have shared a personal tragedy.
I give them my deepest sympathy.

This book would not have been possible without my wonderful
wife, Melody. Her encouragement, graphic art skills and determination to get me to write this book deserve much
more than a thank you.

The last people I would like to thank are those medical professionals who have contributed to our understanding of G6PDD. I
am in hopes that a few will read this book and become inspired to
learn more and do more for us "canaries in the coal mine".

"May I see the day when all babies are screened for
G6PDD and every doctor knows the truth
about living with G6PDD."

-Dale R. Baker

CHAPTER 1

My Story

In 1956, when I was eight years old, our family had just got out of church . After getting into the car I became aware that I wasn't feeling very well. I told my mother, who was sitting on the front passenger's side of the car and she immediately turned around and pulled my lower eyelid down so she could see the underside. She was looking for paleness and she found it. She told my father to get me to the hospital, quickly.

The hospital was thirty miles from us, but my father made the trip in short order. Even so, when we arrived at the hospital I was so weak that I was unable to walk and my father carried me into the hospital.

That was the year that researchers discovered G6PD deficiency, so at that time the doctors knew nothing about G6PDD but my mother did. (Carson 1956, Marshall 2012) She also knew what to do as she got in the doctor's face and told him to give me blood and do it immediately. My father, who was a federal police officer, backed her up and the doctor chose to honor my mother's request. It saved my life.

The family blood disease

We knew G6PDD as "the family blood disease," and had dealt with it for generations. Members of my family had died or had been institutionalized due to what is now known as kernicterus, which was caused by extreme jaundice. (Kernicterus 2013, Washington, 1995) They had also died of iron poisoning, among other problems. My family knew a lot about G6PDD, but unfortunately, not enough. It took until the turn of the century for me to learn that what my mother had been taught was not all true.

My mother's knowledge came mostly from experience. However, much of what she knew came from my family's involvement with Dr. Beutler, who was doing research on G6PDD in Illinois where most of my family lived. My mother made me memorize "the family blood disease's" new name: Familial Congenital Nonspherocytic Hemolytic Anemia Glucose 6 Phosphate Dehydrogenase Deficiency.

Most of you will recognize the last part of the name as G6PD deficiency. But what on earth does the first part mean? These days it is known as chronic nonspherocytic hemolytic anemia or CNSHA. It is what makes Class I G6PDD different from Class II. It means that those who have it are always hemolyzing, whether they come into contact with a G6PDD trigger or not.

Hemolysis in babies with G6PDD

When a baby hemolyzes right after birth it can be life threatening, as an infant's liver and other organs are immature and cannot process the toxins that enter the blood stream when this happens. The baby's body also has not learned to make more than a normal amount of RBCs to compensate for their loss. This is often the first sign that the baby has inherited the mutated gene that causes G6PDD. Unless the doctors or parents are aware of all the "triggers" and remove them, the baby could die. (Dhillon 2008, Nicole 2000)

One reason hemolysis is so critical for babies is that when RBCs die, they release bilirubin into the blood stream which turns the baby yellow. This is called jaundice. The reason it is a big deal is that bilirubin is toxic to nerves. If the concentration of bilirubin becomes high enough, it can cause irreversible brain damage (kernicterus). Older children and adults with mature livers can get rid of this increase in bilirubin, but a newborn baby cannot. The baby must get treatment as quickly as possible. Hospitals treat it by either putting the baby under ultraviolet light which helps the body process the bilirubin much faster or, in extreme cases, they give the baby a blood replacement transfusion. (Jaundice and Kernicterus Symptoms 2013))

Learning about triggers

Over the years, people have asked me to help them find a way to stop their baby from hemolyzing when their doctors are unsuccessful. So far my suggestions have always helped. It isn't so difficult, but you do have to accept the fact that there are other things which can cause hemolysis besides a few drugs, moth balls and fava beans.

Through helping parents all around the world, I have found that removing everything on the avoid lists from a child's diet (and from the mother's diet if they are nursing) helped the child get better. (See Chapters 7, 9, 10 and 11) For moms who cannot nurse their babies, it is a challenge, as I have yet to find a baby formula that doesn't contain foods that are on the contraindicated list for people with G6PDD.

Of course, moth balls, fingernail polish and remover, paint and other things with petrochemicals in them all have to go. Moth balls are especially toxic. Exposure to them at all (even if they are still in their wrappers) can cause hemolysis. Experts around the world are restricting their use. (Alderson 2008, Tarnow-Mordi 2011)

Fava beans are another major food source to avoid, as are all legumes. There have been reports of people hemolyzing just by walking past a field of fava beans.

Vitamin K shots, very commonly given at birth, also have been reported to cause severe hemolysis and death of G6PDD babies. Even though the research is not conclusive that Vitamin K (phytonadione) is the culprit, manufacturers have printed warning labels saying that the Vitamin K shot can be deadly in 'rare' cases, especially for those with G6PDD. (VITAMIN K[1] (phytonadione) Injection 2011) The main problem here is that babies are given the Vitamin K shot routinely right after birth, which means that babies are not even tested for G6PDD until AFTER they get the Vitamin K shot. (There are safer options which are discussed in Chapter 4: "Caring for Babies with G6PD Deficiency.")

So here's the problem: If parents do not know they are G6PDD, or have no clue that their baby may have inherited this genetic enzyme deficiency, how are they going to know what to do, or watch for, before, during and after their baby's birth? Many times the problem isn't diagnosed for weeks, months or even years later. In the meantime, the baby suffers and in some cases dies or is severely handicapped. According to the many parents who have shared their stories with me over the past six years, many of them did not learn about G6PDD until their newborn baby suffered unnecessarily from severe anemia, jaundice and sometimes death. What a tragic, and totally preventable, outcome of ignorance.

How our bodies learn to compensate

The good news is that as a child grows, he or she will become less susceptible to the consequences of hemolysis. The body quickly learns to compensate by making more RBCs than a non-affected person. Organs like the liver and spleen become better at removing the waste products of hemolysis. Symptoms will become less noticeable over time. But those organs are still working harder and they need extra resources to keep up with the increased "work load."

A person with G6PDD needs extra resources to make RBCs and clean up the dead ones. When they are not supplied, the body's ability to do its job is diminished. Eating foods high in the vitamins necessary to build RBCs is necessary for the body keep up with the increased demand.

Not all people with G6PDD have the severe symptoms described above. Some people have no noticeable symptoms for years or attribute them to other things, and then one day they get an infection or take a contraindicated drug, and suddenly they are in trouble.

My mother was asymptomatic, or at least we thought she was. But as I look back on her life I recognize the symptoms of G6PDD. She would get exhausted at times for example. I can't help but think that if I had known then what I know now, she would have lived a healthier life and perhaps still be with us today.

As I continue to interact with the hundreds of people who visit the website, write or call me every day with their stories, I have learned that no matter what class of G6PDD people may have inherited the right circumstances, can suddenly cause them to become very ill, and compromise their quality of life due to the effects of chronic hemolysis. As with any disease, the people who have the most severe reactions teach the others how to manage it.

Notes:

CHAPTER 2

How G6PD Deficiency Was Discovered

Favism gets a new name

In the mid 1900's drug companies noticed that some people given primaquine, a drug used to treat malaria, became very anemic. The armed forces commissioned a team of scientists to find out why. In 1956, Dr. Carson's team published the results of their research which identified an enzyme deficiency as the cause (Carson 1956). This inherited enzyme deficiency was called "Glucose 6 Phosphate Dehydrogenase Deficiency", or G6PD deficiency (G6PDD). It was a new name for a very old condition known as Favism (named after the fava bean), which also caused anemia when consumed by some people.

Dr. Beutler also became involved in G6PDD research and answered questions about varying degrees of hemolysis, X chromosome inactivation, and many other things. These early researchers have provided the backbone of subsequent research. G6PDD is the most common enzyme deficiency in the world, and it's prevalence varies significantly from region to region. Most research articles claim that G6PDD affects approximately 400 million people. However, according to Devi (2010), G6PDD affects a total of 10% of the population, which in todays world, would be approximately 700 million people.

It is called G6PD deficiency because a mutated gene on the X chromosome responsible for the production of the glucose 6 phosphate dehydrogenase (G6PD) enzyme does not produce enough. According to Dr. Staton, an Associate Professor of Medicine at Harvard Medical School, "G6PD is central to the health of all cells being essential for cell survival." (2013) Other research shows that a shortage of G6PD in the body contributes to an increase in hyperglycemia and hypertension. The most well known function of the G6PD enzyme is to work as a co-enzyme in the creation of substances that reduce oxidative stress (free radicals in the blood stream). A deficiency of G6PD will impede the process of turning glutathione into reduced glutathione (GHS), the body's big-gun antioxidant. Because GHS is able to absorb free radicals, it protects the red blood cell from oxidative stress damage and death. Other cells have alternate ways to protect themselves against these destructive free radicals. RBCs do not and are therefore vulnerable to damage (hemolysis) by drugs, food, infections and other substances that cause oxidative stress. (Elyassi 2009)

The dangerous effects of outdated information

Depending on our health, the stress our bodies are under, and other environmental issues we are dealing with, hemolysis caused by oxidative stress ranges from mild to very severe. In some cases, RBC loss is so sudden that a blood transfusion is necessary to prevent death.(Hershko 2011)

In most all cases, one can control hemolysis by simply avoiding the oxidative stress in the first place. People with G6PDD can do that by living a healthier lifestyle and by carefully avoiding the many drugs, foods and other substances known as "triggers" that contribute to it. Unfortunately, the majority of people who suffer from the ill effects G6PDD are those who do not know they have it, and therefore do not know why they suffer from poor health. Then there are those who are diagnosed, but still do not know how to avoid potential health risks because the medical profession largely ignores G6PDD.

Many of the claims made in the first research documents were proven to be false, but they still persist in some medical schools and Online. Most of the doctors I have seen either have never heard of G6PDD or have misconceptions about it. Some of these misconceptions have resulted in death, brain damage or spastic cerebral palsy. Fortunately, doctors and other medical professionals are beginning to learn more about G6PDD and take it more seriously.

The common belief of doctors who have heard of G6PDD is "It is no big deal. Just avoid a few drugs, fava beans and mothballs and you'll be fine. Even if you do have severe hemolysis, you can go to the hospital and get a blood transfusion and you will be fine". In today's world, getting a blood transfusion can be very dangerous. Blood transfusions spread AIDS and other diseases and can have other worse consequences. For example, recently a doctor took a common drug, hemolyzed and had to have blood. A rare complication called TRALI resulted from the transfusion. For him, it was fatal. Another doctor, a friend of the family, convinced his daughters to get tested for G6PD. They tested positive. Had the doctor known he had G6PDD, he would not have taken the drug and his daughters would not be fatherless. (Silliman 2002)

G6PDD is not a recessive trait

The cause of G6PDD is a mutated gene on the X chromosome. In simple terms, women pass the condition to their sons and daughters, and men pass it to their daughters. When first discovered, researchers thought that G6PDD was a recessive trait. That is significant only for women, as men have only one X chromosome, but women have two. If the G6PDD gene only affects one of the X chromosomes, researchers mistakenly thought that the good X chromosome would compensate for the affected one and the woman would be asymptomatic. Two un-related research projects have since proven this false.

In women with only one affected X chromosome, often erroneously called carriers, something called lyonization results. (See Chapter 8: G6PDD Inheritance.) This process occurs very early in an embryo's life. Each cell randomly chooses one of the X chromosomes to deactivate and passes that choice to its progeny. This means that some of her RBCs will have G6PDD and some will not. How many will have the G6PDD gene is a random number from none to all of them. Most women will fall somewhere in the middle. The affected RBCs will die when exposed to oxidative stress. Since only about half of her RBCs have this trait, hemolysis will be less severe than someone who has all of their RBCs affected, but hemolysis in lesser amounts is still a problem. (See Chapter 5: G6PD Deficiency and Women for further discussion.)

Health risks associated with G6PDD

The body must dispose of dead RBCs and make new ones. This process requires resources and has some adverse effects on the body. Chronic hemolysis can cause several problems, including; enlarged bones, clogging of the veins in the eyes, over worked heart, overly stressed kidneys, diabetes, spleen and liver problems and accelerated vitamin use. Other medical conditions are exacerbated and recovery is slower. (Gaskin 2001, Heymann 2012, Mutoni 2007, Staton 2013, Zang 2009)

The good news is that when people with G6PDD stay away from all causes of oxidative stress and follow nutrition practices that restore lost resources, they are less prone to some cancers and aging. (Fulghesu 2011) People unaffected by G6PDD can also benefit from these same practices. Some call us "the canaries in the coal mine" because oxidative stress affects us quicker than it does others, but we are all affected in some way eventually.

Is there a cure for G6PDD?

Many people over the years have asked me if there is a cure for G6PDD. The answer is no, but you can control it... not with drugs or therapy, but by simply staying away from the things that cause oxidative stress (triggers).

Some people get upset due to the number of foods and drugs that are triggers, but there are people with allergies who must avoid the things that cause them. Diabetics must avoid carbohydrates. G6PDD is just another condition that requires some food avoidance. Fortunately, avoiding triggers is good for everyone and helps us to have less susceptibility to other nasty human ailments, like cancer and aging.

CHAPTER 3

Hemolytic Anemia

Hemolysis is the premature destruction of red blood cells (RBCs) that can lead to hemolytic anemia when the bone marrow cannot compensate for the loss of RBCs. Normally, RBCs live between 90 and 120 days, so about 1% of RBCs die each day. But during hemolysis, we can lose most of our RBCs very quickly.

Causes of hemolytic anemia

A number of things can cause hemolytic anemia. Some acquired and others inherited. For those with G6PDD, oxidative stress can cause the premature destruction of RBCs due to the lack of an enzyme called reduced glutathione, which G6PD helps to produce. Certain drugs, foods and other substances are contraindicated because they have been known to cause varying degrees of oxidative stress, which causes RBCs to die prematurely. (Wright 1996, Rees 1993)

Flu, colds, and some other infections can also cause hemolysis, which can sometimes be very severe, or even deadly, especially in infants and small children or when combined with other causes of hemolysis. Because infections put an additional strain on our already compromised immune system due to the lack of G6PD, infections increase the risk of hemolysis. If people then take drugs that are contra-indicated to relieve their symptoms, there are now two forces that are causing increased RBC death. Depending on the health, age, the type of infection, variant and Class of the G6PDD patient, the situation has the potential of becoming critical very quickly. (Ho 2007)

People with Class I G6PD Deficiency suffer from chronic non-spherocytic hemolytic anemia (CNSHA) which means the body is always in some state of hemolysis. Even though Class I is considered relatively rare, it is associated with over 61 variants of G6PDD. (Fiorelli 2000, McKusick 1987)

Degrees of hemolytic anemia

Hemolysis can be quite subtle, or it can be severe enough to be life threatening. One of the things RBCs do is carry oxygen to other cells in our bodies. When enough of them die, the body will have no means of getting oxygen to the other cells. Unless the patient gets immediate medical attention, the result is death. The usual treatment for severe hemolysis is a transfusion of whole blood, but this also has health risks. In any case, it is always best to avoid the triggers that have the potential of causing even mild hemolytic anemia in the first place. (Silliman 2002)

Symptoms of hemolytic anemia

When RBCs undergo hemolysis, or die, the person will have hemolytic anemia. The typical signs and symptoms of hemolytic anemia are:

- abnormal paleness or lack of color of the skin or underside of eyelids
- grayish-blue coloring to fingernails or tongue

- jaundice, or yellowing of the skin, eyes, and mouth

- fever

- dizziness

- confusion

- headache

- weakness

- intolerance of physical activity

- difficulty breathing

- tea-colored urine

- rapid or strong heart beats (tachycardia)

- heart murmur

- abdominal or back pain or both

(Staff, Mayo Clinic. "Anemia" 2013)

Can mild hemolysis be dangerous?

This is always a difficult concept for people to accept, as I get many comments from people who question whether or not they should avoid some of the foods on the contraindicated list if they are eating those items on a regular basis and they don't notice any of the symptoms of hemolysis as listed above. My answer is that if they eat something and see no immediate negative effects, it's easy to think that it's okay to eat that food. Unfortunately, ALL foods, which cause oxidative stress, cause RBCs to die prematurely. If they eat one thing that causes just a little hemolysis and then eat another, the cumulative effect is more than a little hemolysis. Increased hemolysis can then become dangerous. If they then contract an infection, or have any stress or trauma in their life, their blood cell count could drop to dangerous levels much faster. For example, what if you get sick with something that causes hemolysis and then take something for it that also causes hemolysis. If you also combine this with poor health or being anemic to begin with, you could find yourself in very serious trouble. ("G6PD" 2013)

I have preached for years that it is imperative that we stay in top-notch health, eat good nutritious food, and exercise, if for no other reason than to protect ourselves from these times in our lives. Personally, I believe anyone diagnosed with G6PDD needs to avoid everything that causes oxidative stress, otherwise they may increase their chances of hemolysis.

Prevention is your best defense

Since G6PDD is a genetic disorder, there is no cure. The best way to avoid the health risks associated with hemolytic anemia is to live a healthy life style (eat healthy foods, get plenty of rest and exercise) and avoid certain drugs and foods and other substances (called "triggers") which are on the contraindicated lists. It is also very important to do your best to eat foods, or take supplements that will replenish the vitamins and minerals necessary to make more RBCs, (See Chapter 9: "Diet Suggestions").

CHAPTER 4

Caring for Babies with G6PD Deficiency

Pregnant and nursing mothers and G6PDD

It is very important that All mothers of G6PDD babies avoid ALL contraindicated substances (triggers) while nursing. If you are pregnant and there is a chance that your baby might inherit G6PDD from either parent, you should also avoid all triggers during your pregnancy. Also, be sure to eat plenty of antioxidants.

What to look for at birth

Research shows that 60% of newborn babies, develop jaundice (yellow skin caused by too much bilirubin in their system), and about 1 in 20 need treatment. (Jaundice and Kernicterus 2013, Jaundice, Newborn 2010;) However, if your baby is a boy or a fully deficient girl with G6PDD, statistics show that the chances of suffering from jaundice is 1.5 times that a baby without G6PDD. (Glucose-6-Phosphate Dehydrogenase Deficiency 2013, Al-Omran 1999, Hussain 2010,) According to a study done in 2010, four out of 8 babies diagnosed with G6PDD were treated for jaundice. (Iglessias) In some regions it is uncommon for a G6PDD baby boy NOT to have a serious hemolytic episode within the first two weeks of life. Partially deficient girls are usually at a lower risk for acute hemolysis.

The increased jaundice is due to RBCs releasing their bilirubin into the baby's blood stream during hemolysis. Because a baby's liver is not able to rid its body of bilirubin fast enough, the bilirubin builds up (hyperbilirubinemia) and causes jaundice. If not treated quickly, it can cause kernicterus (permanent brain damage) or death. The usual treatment is to place the baby under special lights or give the baby a blood transfusion. The good news, barring other complications, these treatments are virtually 100% effective in keeping babies out of danger, as long as all triggers are removed from the G6PDD baby's environment. (Frank 2005, Moiz 2012)

Even though the research is controversial, hospitals routinely give newborns Vitamin K shots immediately after birth, as they believe it prevents internal bleeding, so the benefits outweigh the risks. (VITAMIN K1 (phytonadione) Injection 2011) What mom's don't know is that if internal bleeding is caused by a Vitamin K deficiency it can largely be avoided by making sure the mother gets plenty of vitamin K in her diet, especially right before birth. There is also evidence that waiting to remove the umbilical cord until after the baby has assimilated the blood in it, and letting the baby nurse immediately, will give him or her the extra blood and clotting enzymes they need until their own reserves of Vitamin K increase naturally in their digestive system. (Rothville 2011)

Feeding your G6PD deficient baby

By far the best milk for a baby with G6PDD is breast milk. If a nursing mom has eaten or taken anything on the avoid list, I recommend that she stop nursing, pump and discard her breast milk until these things are no longer present in her milk.

Unfortunately, not all mothers can breast feed, which can complicate matters for a G6PDD baby. We have researched every baby formula we know about and ALL of them have contraindicated substances in them... usually soy or ascorbic acid, or both. If you are unable to breastfeed your baby, we recommend making your own baby formula from fresh goat's milk as an alternative. (See: http://www.rockwellnutrition.com/Can-I-use-Goat-Milk-instead-of-infant-formula_ep_92-1.html)

If your physician recommends vitamins, be sure the vitamins are from a natural food source. Vitamins that do not come from a natural food source are generally not as safe. Please be cautious about introducing new foods and vitamins to your baby, as research shows that mother's milk provides sufficient nutrition for the first six to eight months of life, or even longer. (Huh 2011) Adding food to your baby's diet does not help them sleep through the night, in fact there is evidence showing that adding foods too early can contribute to your baby becoming an obese toddler. (Macknin 1989)

If you are unable to get fresh (or even canned) goat's milk then the next best formula would be a home-made formula from fresh (or canned) cow's milk. Mothers of babies who are lactose intolerant have developed very nutritious formulas using rice milk. (See: http://jennpike.wordpress.com/2010/01/09/home-made-rice-milk-based-infant-formula) One good thing about rice milk, is that if you can't find it in stores, you can make your own. (See: http://www.justmommies.com/blog/2011/10/make-your-own-rice-milk) For additional information, recipes and link at the end of this chapter or visit g6pddeficiency.org.

Some good first foods for G6PD deficient babies

The best solid foods for your baby are those that you prepare yourself from fresh ingredients. It takes a little more preparation, but your own mashed or blended foods are healthier and better tasting. If you wait to introduce solid food until your baby is older, they can learn to feed themselves finger foods like soft cooked veggies or fruits. However, if there are times where you need the convenience of purchasing baby food from the store, be sure to check the ingredients carefully for soy products. Many times, soy is disguised as lecithin or vegetable broth.

First foods should be as a single ingredient. Another reason that homemade foods are MUCH better is you have total control over the ingredients. Here are some examples.

Rice cereal has been a staple first food for a long time. To make it, simply grind cooked organic whole grain rice in a blender or food processor and thin with some breast milk or goat's milk.

Avocados and bananas are also great first foods and they are simple to prepare and contain foliate, which they need for blood production. Just remove the meat and mash with a fork. Add breast milk or goat's milk to thin or rice cereal to thicken.

Pears, yams/sweet potatoes and winter squash can be prepared by steaming or baking until tender and then processing in a blender or food processor. Add a bit of breast milk or goat's milk to thin or rice cereal to thicken. Be sure to cool to warm before serving.

Apples can be made into applesauce by peeling, coring and cutting into chunks. Just cover with water and boil until soft. Be sure to stir often and do not use aluminum pans. Drain the apples, reserving water, and puree. Add some of the reserved water to thin or rice cereal to thicken. Serve slightly warm. Canned applesauce is acceptable if it contains apples and water and nothing else.

- - - - -

For recipes and creative preparation tips visit: http://umaine.edu/publications/4309e/

For recipes and additional information from moms whose babies have G6PDD check out these web articles:

"Baby Food and G6PD Deficiency" (http://www.homemade-baby-food-recipes.com/baby-food-and-g6pd-deficiency.html).

"Foods for a Baby With G6PD Deficiency" (http://www.homemade-baby-food-recipes.com/foods-for-a-baby-with-G6PD-deficiency.html)

CHAPTER 5

G6PD Deficiency and Women

Women who are G6PD deficient are the most affected by the myths and erroneous assumptions that have been passed around for more than six decades. Poorly researched articles whose authors have based their conclusions on research that has already been proven false propagated these outdated "facts". These articles were (and still are) used to develop a hypothesis for other articles and research papers, and the assumptions soon became "well knows facts"... which are taught as such in medical schools world wide. To make matters even worse, along comes the Internet which has a way of passing around these erroneous, outdated facts at lightening speed. However, thanks to a few researchers, and other interested individuals (who have actually done their homework) more accurate information regarding the prevalence and symptoms of individuals with G6PDD is finally making it's way to the surface.

Blood tests for G6PDD

The advent of blood tests, like the G6PD quantitative test, are giving doctors a more accurate tool to diagnose women who are only partially deficient. These women were hemolyzing when exposed to drugs and other triggers, but were either misdiagnosed or accused of being hypochondriacs. Using the old florescence test the ratio of boys to girls who have G6PDD is 4 : 1.5 respectively. This is statistically impossible (Reclos, et al 2000)

Both boys and girls have an equal chance of inheriting G6PDD from their mother. So the same number of boys and girls should have G6PDD if this was the only way to inherit the enzymeopathy. However, only girls can inherit G6PDD from their father. Now the number of affected girls should be greater than boys. The actual ratio turns out to be 5.5 girls to 4 boys. In other words, the florescence test misses 75% of positive girls.

Even today, because there are now over 400 known variants, and the prevalence for G6PDD can vary from 1% to over 50% from race to race, and region to region, doctors are finding it very frustrating when trying to learn better ways of recognizing the symptoms, diagnosing, and treating their patients. If you look on the Internet, even those organizations who claim to be experts on the subject disagree on what individuals need to do to minimize the health risks for those with G6PDD.

Here are some of the more common myths that involve women with G6PDD:

Myth #1: More men are G6PDD than women.

For reasons stated above, the actual statistics show that slightly more women than men have G6PDD.

Myth #2: Women who have G6PDD are asymptomatic (do not hemolyze).

Because lower levels of hemolysis are sometimes very difficult to detect, it contributes to the myth that women are unaffected. This was proven wrong by two different research teams working independently. One of the teams was headed by Dr. Beutler, who spent over 50 years studying G6PDD. He was puzzled by a female patient who was considered to be only a "carrier" as she only had one X-chromosome that was affected, yet when exposed to contraindicated substances, she would hemolyze so quickly that she had to be given transfusions to save her life. Until this point in time, he did not think it was possible for partially deficient women to hemolyze. With the help of the research work of Dr. Judy Lyon, he was able to understand why this was possible. (Beutler 1962)

Partially deficient vs. fully deficient

Women who have G6PDD come in two categories: Either with one or both X chromosomes affected. If both are affected, they are considered fully deficient and have symptoms like men. The other group, with only one affected X chromosome (partially deficient) vary in severity from mild to severe based on Lyonization.

Lyonization is a process of selecting which X chromosome will be deactivated in a cell. It is a random process and happens early in an embryo's life. Each cell chooses an X-chromosome to deactivate and passes this choice to its progeny. How many choose to deactivate the X chromosome affected by G6PDD determines how deficient the woman will be. ("X-chromosome inactivation" 2013)

Let's look at it in a simpler way: If half of the RBCs have the good X chromosome deactivated, then half of her RBCs will be fully deficient and half will be unaffected. When she comes into contact with a trigger, half of her blood cells will react and half will not. This ratio is completely random and can vary from only a small portion of RBCs affected to most of them affected. The resulting hemolysis from triggers will be small to large respectively. So, women are affected by triggers, but how much depends on the results of Lyonization.

The dangers of inaccurate testing for G6PDD

The reason that women in general have been misdiagnosed, is that most G6PDD tests return a false negative for women with one affected X chromosome. (Reclos, Katzidakis, Shculpis 2000) But it is not only her health that is being negatively affected. The bad news is that if she has been misdiagnosed and thinks that she does not have G6PDD, she won't know that she has a 50% chance of passing her affected X chromosome to her son. Her doctor will not be aware of the precautions to avoid contraindicated foods and drugs, especially if she finds out she is going to have a boy. This could, and does, cause the baby unnecessary health risks, as babies with G6PDD are at much higher risk of suffering from the ill effects of neonatal jaundice caused by acute hemolysis. (Washington 1995)

The good news is that more accurate testing procedures are now being implemented. Until recently (depending on how and when the test given), if the woman was recovering from a recent hemolytic episode the test would not show that any of her blood cells were deficient, as they had all died and the test would produce a false negative. Also the cutoff from the old florescent test was too high to find partially deficient females. (Redos et al. 2013)

Do women need to avoid triggers? Yes. They should avoid triggers just like men, even though lower levels of hemolysis are difficult to detect. Even though the resulting hemolysis is, as a rule, less than that of a fully deficient woman or a man, any hemolysis over time can lead to other health problems and can cause other illnesses to be more severe.

CHAPTER 6

G6PD Deficiency & Resistance To Malaria

G6PD deficiency is said to provide resistance against malaria infection. This concept was first examined after scientists noticed a correlation between areas of the world where G6PDD is prevalent and regions where malaria is endemic. It has even been suggested that the G6PDD gene mutation is nature's way of providing the body with resistance against malaria. This hypothesis is understandable since the discovery of G6PDD as a genetic disorder was partially fueled by the reaction of G6PDD patients to anti-malarials such as Primaquine and quinine. However, the research does not take into account that even though patients with G6PDD have a greater chance of survival, because their symptoms are atypical, their illnesses are not reported as malaria, especially in underdeveloped countries where malaria is most prevalent.

How malaria infects our bodies

Malaria is transmitted to humans by mosquitoes infected with a parasite. These parasites incubate in the liver. Most types of malaria will make a person very sick within a week to ten days. However, there are some types that will remain dormant for up to four years before they will start reproducing and causing their host to become ill. When the malaria parasites are mature enough to be released into the blood stream, they will then infect RBCs. The parasites continue to grow and replicate in the RBCs for 10 to 14 days until the RBCs burst and several poisons created by the malaria parasite are released into the blood stream, which causes the high fever, chills and sweats.

Malaria parasites and G6PD deficient RBCs

Malaria parasites cannot thrive in immature RBCs. Because hemolysis affects mature RBCs more readily there are fewer of them to host malaria parasites. When an infected RBC dies before the parasite has matured, the malaria parasite dies as well and it does not have the chance to produce the poisons. Because of this, the typical symptoms do not usually manifest themselves in G6PDD patients. So it is possible that atypical symptoms could make malaria more difficult to diagnose and account for the belief that it is less prevalent in G6PDD patients. Malaria can still sequester in the liver of a G6PDD host, however. The dangerous part is two fold: a G6PDD patient can die or become very ill from hemolysis; G6PDD patients cannot take anti-malarials. Some malaria types start making their own G6PD after a few cycles which nullifies having G6PDD in the first place. If you are a female, and only one of your X chromosomes is G6PD deficient, you may not have any resistance to malaria at all. Though malaria can't thrive in G6PDD blood cells, it takes severe hemolysis to kill it. Primaquine is the major drug to kill malaria that has sequestered in the liver, yet people with G6PDD cannot take it as it increases hemolysis (Bhalla 2004).

It is a fallacy to say that G6PDD offers a protection against malaria. Here is why:

1. If that were true, then why would the United States armed forces test all of their recruits for G6PDD?

2. If G6PDD recruits have a resistance to malaria then why are they must all soldiers with G6PDD be issued a medical alert dog tag? (United States of America 2008).

This rumor has been propagated only because the prevalence of people with G6PDD is much higher in regions where malaria is present, and in many cases it has been shown that the most deadly strain of infested parasites cannot survive as well in a few variants of fully deficient people. Even though both past and present research show that there are other factors, such as genetic drift, that could account for the higher incidence of people with G6PDD in those areas, most researchers are still presenting this hypothesis as fact. ("G6PD Deficiency Protects against Severe Malaria" 2013, Seidlein 2013, McKusik 2013)

The truth is, people with G6PDD get malaria just as easily as everyone else. In fact G6PDD was discovered because the United States armed forces wanted to find out why some of their recruits would hemolyze when given Primaquine to treat them for malaria. Even now, all of the anti-malarials listed by the Center for Disease Control (CDC) are contraindicated, except Doxycycline, which cannot be taken by pregnant women or children under the age of eight.

Center for Disease Control precautions against mosquitoe bites

Because people with G6PDD can get malaria just as easily as everyone else, and because people with G6PDD cannot take the most effective medicines for malaria, we strongly advise you to take the following precautions when visiting malaria-endemic areas:

- Use natural repellents and insecticides on outside of clothing and avoid contact with skin as much as possible. Use light applications and allow clothing to dry before use. Avoid Deet, petrochemicals and chemicals derived from petrochemicals. We recommend not using of aerosols.

• It would be best to try repellents in small amounts before visiting malaria-endemic areas to make sure hemolysis does not occur from their use.

- - - - -

A letter from Dr. Ogundu concerning malaria:

"G6pdd conferring immunity against malaria is a myth, not just any myth but a dangerous one. Most may remember I posted the fact that I almost met my maker in March 2011 when I came down with Malaria during my visits to sub-Saharan Africa. So we do get them. Ask those in military. They have the statistics. This is what happens to us:

Plasmodium species, of which Falciparum is most ubiquitous, vector is mosquito and only replicates inside matured erythrocytes, i.e. RBCs. This is where the confusion started. As we know, we with g6pdd are blessed with fragile RBCs. Therefore, as our matured RBCs get inoculated with this parasite they do what they do best, hemolyze and in doing this destroys the parasite with self since the parasite can't live in blood stream outside the RBC. The problem is our body fights better by doing what most of the drugs are intended to do but if prolonged and severe an attack, our hemolysis is more threatening. This may explain why malaria is dubbed the "world's most dangerous infectious disease," at a globally 3.3 billion at risk mosquito-borne disease, it claims over a million lives annually but, read this, over half are noted where g6pdd is endemic. The good news is the lack of g6pd allows early destruction of our RBCs so that a bad infestation won't take hold as we immediately build up on uninfectable reticulocytes. This is our saving grace. However, the other side of the coin, with that early sequestration we are anemic, bilirubin start building up and if you have not paid attention to your health and followed Dale's health catechism, you are already behind the eight ball. Borderline or any state of anemia is not where you want to be if attacked by malaria.

Also, one of the problems is finding a non-homicidal drug for people with g6pdd. Most of the old ones are no-nos. Some say take in smaller doses. Take it from this guinea pig, don't try it on your own.

Presently, there are newer drugs. Part of the testing is using our blood for testing. We are the ideal canaries in this coal mine.

1. Malarone is a combo drug best against P. falciparum, acts at liver stage and blood level. Our problem is atovaquone may be judiciously taken but the other part of the combo, proguanil causes hematuria in some people. To me this says stay away if you tend to hemolyze.

2. Tafenoquine is a long acting 8-amino quinoline with half life in weeks not hours. Stay far away from this drug. It is one that they actually stated: Do not give in presence of g6pdd.

3. Lariam and Fansidar cause oxidant-induced hemolytic anemia with methemoglobinemia. Stay away from these.

4. Clindamycin (Dalacin) although causes blood dyscracia, liver damage and colitis may work but need high dose that exposes one to colitis.

5. Doxycycline under Vibramycin, Vibra tabs, Doryxy. Can cause blood dyscrias, rarely esophageal ulcers. Commonly Candida overgrowth in women and sensitivity to sunlight.

6. Azithromycin (G.I upsets)

7. Halofantrine is quinine and mefloquine in fancy name and suit. Stay far away!

8. Pyronaridine is the new drug from China and for your health it is same as chloroquine.

9. Artemisin is a derivative of Qmghaosu. It is said to be safe for us

with g6pdd BUT, until they explain about the controversial brain tumors in those poor rodents and the neurotoxicity I won't be anywhere near it.

Having said all these, my take home is do your research. For me, I take precaution against malaria because when we do come down with it, it's not pretty. I use my home made spray, prevention therapy of doxycycline 100mg daily and, if I come down with it I go for Azithhromycin. Although some infectious disease experts will opt for doubling same doxycycline 100mg twice a day for 7days. Women if you do, get monistat or eat plain cultured yogurt to ward off the yeast that will come. Of course, I always have my net to sleep in and bright PJ's.

Lastly, there is a new baby added for prevention, the Zero-Vector Durable Lining (DL) by DART. It is a combo of insecticidal nets plus indoor residual spraying(IRS) that lasts 3 years. The nets are said to be safe. And made from woven thick polyethylene panels that are treated with Deltametrin (a WHO recommended insecticide said to be safe). Unfortunately, no one could give me a printable answer regarding Deltametrin's safety in g6pdd so I did my own digging. These are what are available, "neurotoxic in humans, found in breast milk, highly toxic to aquatic life(fish). No mention of g6pdd effect. Didn't expect one and they didn't disappoint. WHO does not see g6pdd as a problem. I agree with them it is not in an ideal environment but, none of in our over chemicalized environment would call it ideal.

Please continue to take precautions against ALL infections. We do poorly with all of them. The best prevention is one I never was exposed to. Stay healthy and remember statistics is number game, when you are that one, percentages don't matter.

G6PDD does not kill. IGNORANCE does."Dr. Ogundu
(This letter was posted on the g6pddeficiency.org forum in 2012)

Notes:

CHAPTER 7

Why We Recommend Avoiding Legumes

There is a lot of controversy about legumes causing hemolysis in G6PD deficient patients. In order to address this issue, I will first address the issue of varying degrees of hemolysis.

Dangers of chronic low level hemolysis

In my experience, the majority of doctors and other medical professionals see hemolysis in G6PDD patients as an all or nothing problem. If you don't hemolyze badly enough to need treatment at a hospital, then you're fine. I strongly disagree with this for the following reasons:

The vast majority of hemolytic events are mild enough for the body to compensate for without intervention. Following this reasoning, it is only logical that hemolysis can happen from very mild to very severe, depending on circumstances such as health, stress, triggers, age, etc.

Many people go for years experiencing hemolysis without knowing it. They can have other health issues that eventually lead to the discovery that they have G6PDD, or, they eventually have a hemolytic crisis. I have received countless emails from people in this last category. Their health issues run from liver, heart, blindness, renal, spleen and chronic yellow color of skin, to death in some cases. These problems can occur from early in life to later in life. Many families discover G6PDD runs in their family only after the needless death or serious illness of a family member, which was caused by G6PDD complications. (Büyükokuroğlu 2002, Wright 2103)

Why red blood cells need G6PD

Now that we know that hemolysis varies in intensity, let's discuss the cause of hemolysis in people with G6PDD. When a red blood cell has sufficient G6PD to complete the pathway to reduce glutathione, the reduced glutathione is then able to neutralize an oxidative substance, rendering it harmless. Those with G6PDD cannot reduce enough glutathione to protect RBCs from damage so the oxidative substance destroys the RBC. It is my opinion that this happens to everyone with G6PDD, regardless of which variant they have.

Because of the health risks involved, what is more important than the variant is the degree (or Class) of G6PDD that you have. (For the purpose of this discussion, both less G6PD and less effective G6PD are synonymous.) One person may have more G6PD than another and therefore that person is able to produce more reduced glutathione to protect RBCs than a person with less G6PD. G6PD also varies in effectiveness. Two people can have the same quantity of G6PD but be in different classes because the G6PD effectiveness is not the same. (Frank 2005)

Legumes and hemolysis

Fava beans or broad beans are listed for all variants of G6PDD in every contraindicated list I have ever seen, yet some G6PDD "experts" insist that some variants do not exhibit Favism. The definition of Favism is a condition that causes hemolysis from exposure to fava beans. I have not yet seen a research paper or other proof as to the exact chemical, or chemicals, in fava beans that cause hemolysis. Convicine and vicine are the generally accepted culprits, but other factors may also contribute to hemolysis. Since convicine and vicine do not exist in other legumes, it does not explain why they also cause hemolysis. Year so, botanists discovered that in the presence of two much iron free radicals cause oxidative stress in the nodules of legumes. If there was more research done, I am wondering if they is a connection with the iron in our bodies that reacts to the legumes, and not the legumes themselves. It's a stretch, but unless there is more research, I suppose we will never know.

Over the past few years, people using hemoglobin meters have shown that many other legumes also cause hemolysis to varying degrees. Again, it is my opinion that all G6PDD people react to these substances, but to varying degrees depending on severity of G6PDD, health, etc. (Valiaveedam 2005)

Because low level hemolysis (or mild hemolysis) is difficult to detect, it is logical that many people who believe they are not reacting to legumes actually are, but not enough to notice. However, low level hemolysis can be very dangerous over time. Our bodies must generate more than the normal amount of RBCs to compensate and dispose of the ones destroyed. This process takes resources needed for healthy bodies. Consequently, we are more susceptible to other diseases and they can be more severe than when we are not undergoing low level hemolysis. ("Misdiagnosis of Anemia." 2013)

To date, medical research is far behind when it come to legumes and G6PDD. Because I have had so much success in stopping hemolysis by avoiding all legumes and products containing them, I recommend that everyone avoid them. I have received thousands of emails, forum posts, and phone calls from people detailing how removing legumes from their diet has helped them and made them feel better. Someday maybe medical research will provide us with more information concerning the exact chemicals in legumes which cause hemolysis.

A letter from a doctor who is also G6PD deficient:

"Fellow travelers:

How much rat poison do you need in your system to poison your body? How often can you expose yourself to it to become immune? If 100 people are exposed to poison, do all die or bleed overtly? And, those who show no clinical signs of poison are they assumed not harmed in any way? It is funny, once you consume poison regardless of clinical presentation; you are treated because we know in the hospital that damage is done regardless. Poisons are dangerous to humans because we lack the specific enzymes to break them down into non-threatening wastes. Likewise, oxidative stressors are our kryptonite. Superman had enough sense to not only stay away from it but bury it out of his existence. He didn't take any chances. None of us are super persons so we must take heed.

Not knowing the facts is one thing, but to be exposed to facts and not consider? That is another thing. There seems to be such arrogance in ignorance that it is baffling. There is quite a big difference between allergy and enzymopathy. Allergy involves the immune system and the body can be re-trained in a method called de-sensitization. On the other hand, enzyme deficiency or dysfunction is what it is, a lack in functionality. When a deficient body is exposed, there is untoward ramification. Seen or unseen the damage happened. Even, the so called partial deficient female (I call insufficiency) definitely suffers damage as well when exposed. However, the response in her case could be likened to a double engine plane in crisis. When one engine is done, unlike its single engine counterpart, it continues to fly and land with the other. Ask, any seasoned pilot, they'll attest that it is not the most desirable situation and that plane got a problem.

As I read along it seems that no matter what likes of Marion, Dale, John and many others advocate, there will be people who prefer to bury their heads in the sand. There is a cliché that g6pdd is not a serious problem. Clichés are myths and like all myths based on prejudicial ignorance and non-facts. The damning danger is that the group most guilty of perpetuating this myth is no other than those sworn keepers of our health, our physicians. This is not only the irony but a disgrace for their lack of investigative curiosity in this genetic dysfunction. Imagine, this is not only one of the 5 most common newborn genetic disorder but, causes more kernicterus (brain damage due to high bilirubin). Yet, in 2011 we continue to quibble on the merit of newborn testing and transformative education.

If I sound angry it is because I am. The stand that you can eat anything except fava beans is not only ignorant but dangerous. I know because the cold earth instead of my mother's warm arms was all that cuddled my 4 male siblings (two same day) after being exposed to a stressor. My vigilance rescued me from my mom's fate when my oldest son took ill after exposure to mothballs. Ironically, my little study has shown that most babies with g6pdd do not naturally like beans but are taught or forced into acquiring the taste. Nature always has a way of protecting us if we pay heed.

Be well."

Dr. Ogundu

(Letter to the g6pddeficiency.org forum, 2011)

CHAPTER 8

G6PD Deficiency Inheritance Chart

A person can inherit G6PDD from one or both parents. It cannot be passed from one person to another in any other way as it is caused by a genetic defect on the X chromosome. Because males inherit their one X chromosome from their mother, males cannot pass their deficient X chromosome to their sons… only their daughters. This is why males can either be G6PD deficient or unaffected. Because females have two X chromosomes, they can inherit a deficient X chromosome from either parent, or both. This is why women can be fully deficient, partially deficient (erroneous known as a 'carrier'), or unaffected.

The G6PD Quantitative Test, like the one that is made by R & D Diagnosiscs, is the only test fo G6PDD that is reliable for both men and women.

The following rules determine the probability of your offspring inheriting G6PD deficiency.

- Father is UNAFFECTED, mother is UNAFFECTED:

- ALL of their children will be UNAFFECTED.

- Father is G6PD DEFICIENT, mother is UNAFFECTED:

- All sons will be UNAFFECTED.

- All daughters will be PARTIALLY DEFICIENT.

- Father is G6PD DEFICIENT, mother is PARTIALLY DEFICIENT (one of her X chromosomes is unaffected):

- Out of two sons, one will be G6PD DEFICIENT and the other will be UNAFFECTED.

- Out of two daughters, one will be PARTIALLY DEFICIENT and the other will be G6PD DEFICIENT.

- Father and mother are G6PD DEFICIENT:

- All children will be G6PD DEFICIENT.

- Father is UNAFFECTED, mother is PARTIALLY DEFICIENT:

- Out of two sons, one will be G6PD DEFICIENT and the other will be UNAFFECTED.

- Out of two daughters, one will be PARTIALLY DEFICIENT, the other UNAFFECTED.

- Father is UNAFFECTED, mother is G6PD DEFICIENT:

- All sons will be G6PD DEFICIENT.

- All daughters will be PARTIALLY DEFICIENT.

Notes:

CHAPTER 9

G6PD Deficiency Diet Suggestions

G6PDD can cause or contribute to the metabolic issues discussed below. You can lessen the impact of these problems through proper diet. This knowledge will help you make informed decisions about the food you eat.

The main object of the G6PDD diet is to provide your body with the nutrients it needs without destroying red blood cells (RBC) in the process. This is especially true if you have Class I (the most severe) G6PDD. You can help your body protect red blood cells by eating antioxidants, providing RBC building nutrients and eating fewer refined carbohydrates. You should also be diligent in avoiding contraindicated drugs, foods and other substances.

Once you understand the ideas presented below, providing a proper diet for anyone with G6PDD is straightforward and can be quite satisfying, delicious and full of variety.

Difficulty digesting fats

Cholesterol is necessary for proper nerve health and without it, we can develop nerve problems such as peripheral neuropathy or multiple sclerosis. Low cholesterol is a problem for some who are G6PD deficient. (Batetta 2002) If you have a problem with low cholesterol, you need a diet rich in fat. Our fats should come from traditional sources (olive oil, animal fat, palm oil and coconut oil) and we should avoid other vegetable fats, especially those that are not expeller pressed. (For a list of foods and cholesterol content, see: http://www.nal.usda.gov/fnic/foodcomp/Data/SR17/wtrank/sr17w601.pdf.)

Susceptibility to diabetes and infections

Since digestion of carbohydrates (especially refined sugar, white flour, high fructose corn syrup, etc) requires G6PD, products containing these ingredients should be limited. Lack of G6PD causes the beta cells, which produce insulin to be smaller, and therefore less effective. This makes people with G6PDD more susceptible to Type 2 diabetes. (Heymann 2002, Zhang 2009)

People with G6PDD need to do everything think they possibly can to avoid getting infections. Infections, just like diabetes, put a huge strain on the body's immune system. This causes free radicals to weaken red blood cells, which in turn increases the rate of hemolysis. If a person with G6PDD is then given contraindicated medications by mistake, the outcome could be deadly. Not only is it important to eat healthy, but it is equally important to get enough rest and excercise to keep the body's immune system in top shape.

Vitamins and antioxidants essential for healthy RBCs

Our vitamins should come from our food as much as possible. Tests to check for adequate levels of vitamins, especially the B vitamins, should be a part of medical checkups. Vitamin B^2, B^6, B^9 and B^{12}, are essential for the formation of new red blood cells. All the B vitamins help the body convert food (carbohydrates) into fuel (glucose), which is used to produce energy. If supplementation is needed , use natural vitamins or increase foods high in these vitamins. Foods with these vitamins include green leafy vegetables such as lettuce, cabbage, spinach, kale, etc. Eat liver and good homemade bone stocks (for soups and sauces) regularly. Most people with G6PDD should supplement their diet with the following vitamins (dose is for an adult) :

Vitamin B^1 (thiamine): 50 mg daily. Helps build strong organs.

Vitamin B^2 (riboflavin): Needed to help the body change vitamin B6 and folate into forms it can use, is important for body growth, reproduction and red cell production. Dairy products, leafy green vegetables, nuts, fruits, organ meats and fish are excellent sources.

Vitamin B^6 (pyridoxine): 50 mg daily. B^6 assists the body in creating antibodies in the immune system. It helps the body maintain normal nerve function and produce hemoglobin within red blood cells. It also helps increase the amount of oxygen carried by hemoglobin. The higher the protein intake, the more need there is for vitamin B^6, to process proteins in the body. Potatoes, bananas, chicken breasts, and pork, are the highest in vitamin B6.

Vitamin B^9 (folate and folic acid): 400 mcg twice daily. Folate occurs naturally in fresh foods, whereas folic acid is the synthetic form found in supplements. Your body needs folate to produce red blood cells, as well as components of the nervous system, and to treat megeloblastic anemia, which is caused by deficiency in folate and vitamin B^{12}. It helps in the formation and creation of DNA and maintaining normal brain function. Folic acid is vital for proper cell growth and development of the embryo. Organ meats, beef jerky, green-leafy vegetables and sunflower seeds are good sources of vitamin B^9. However, it is easily destroyed by overcooking.

Vitamin B^{12} (cobalamin): 500 mcg twice daily. This vitamin is important for metabolism. It helps in the formation of red blood cells and in the maintenance of the central nervous system. Vitamin B^{12} is the one vitamin that is available only from fish, poultry, meat or dairy sources in food.

Vitamin E: 400 iu twice daily. Vitamins A, D, E, & K are in fat. Reduced fat milk, for example, has to be fortified with vitamin D, while whole milk does not. We do not recommend diets high in fat.

However, we do suggest a diet with a reasonable amount of fats so that these vitamins can be obtained naturally. If you are concerned about your cholesterol levels, the July 2009 issue of the Harvard Health Letter suggests that saturated and trans fats have a much bigger affect on blood cholesterol levels. In Chapter 2: Converting Recipes, is a list of acceptable fats, and ways to use them in your cooking.

NAC (N-acetyl-cysteine): 400 mg twice daily. Boosts glutathione and is a powerful antioxidant. (See "The Better Brain Book" by Dr. David Perlmutter)

Citric acid vs. ascorbic acid

Vitamin C (citric acid): This is one of the most important of all vitamins. It protects our body's tissue from the damage of oxidation. Free radicals, which are potentially damaging by-products of the body's metabolism, can cause cell damage that may contribute to the development of cardiovascular disease and cancer. Scientist have found Vitamin C to be an effective antiviral agent. The natural variety found in fruits and vegetables does not cause a problem for those with G6PDD, but the artificially produced ascorbic acid does as it increases the bioavailablty of iron. can be dangerous for G6PDD as chronic hemolysis already increases iron in the blood stream. (See Chapter 11: "Foods to Avoid" for more information)

Overall best sources of antioxidants

In 2002, Brent Halvorsen from the Institute for Nutrition Research, Faculty of Medicine, University of Oslo, in Blindern, Norway, states, "With the data of this report, it is possible for the first time to make a comprehensive calculation of the total intake of antioxidants by an individual and to test the hypothesis that total dietary antioxidants have a protective role in oxidative stress related pathogenesis [...] Our results demonstrated that there is more than a 1000-fold difference among total antioxidants in various dietary plants. Plants that contain most antioxidants included members of several families, such as Rosaceae (dog rose, sour cherry, blackberry, strawberry, raspberry), Empetraceae (crowberry), Ericaceae (blueberry), Grossulariaceae (black currant), Juglandaceae (walnut), Asteraceae (sunflower seed), Punicaceae (pomegranate) and Zingiberaceae (ginger)."[1]

The following is a ranked list by individual plant group, with the highest antioxidant value first. It is a ranked list by individual plant groups and is available Online. (Journal of Nutrition, Halvorsen 2002 <http://jn.nutrition.org/content/132/3/461.full.pdf+html>)

(Note: This is not a complete list. There are additional food sources of antioxidants not analyzed in this study.)

Berries

Dog rose

Crowberry

Bilberry/wild blueberry

Black currant

Sour cherry

Strawberry

Blueberry

Cranberry

Raspberry

Cloudberry

---

1   Most of the information in the antioxidant section came from the University of Maryland's nutrition web pages. (Source: http://www.umm.edu/search-results.htm?q=vitamins)

Ranked List of Foods High in Antioxidants

Fruit

Pomegranate

Grape

Orange

Plum

Pineapple

Lemon

Dates

Kiwi

Clementine

Grapefruit

Nuts, seeds, and dried fruit

Walnuts

Sunflower seeds

Apricots

Prunes

Vegetables

Kale

Chili pepper

Red cabbage

Peppers

Parsley

Artichoke

Brussels Sprouts

Spinach

Cereals

Barley

Millet

Oats

Corn

Roots and Tubers

Ginger

Red Beets

Other Antioxidants

Adding ingredients to your diet that are rich in vitamins and nutrients to your homemade dishes will provide much-needed antioxidants, as well as the building blocks the body needs to create new red blood cells. For example, nutrient rich spinach or mild squash can be added to eggs, meatloaf, soups, while affecting the taste very little. You can chop these, and other vegetables, so small that they look like an herb so people don't suspect you are feeding them a healthier diet. (We even add a little to our smoothies.) Great for getting around picky eaters. Here are a few ideas taken from the book "Staying Healthy with G6PD Deficiency":

1. Broccoli and other green vegetables – You knew these were good for you because your mother told you so! They can be eaten cooked or raw and added to soups, salads and even your main dish.

2. Tomatoes – contain lycopene, a relatively rare member of the carotenoid family, also found in pink grapefruit and twice as powerful as beta-carotene. Studies have shown that men who eat more tomatoes or tomato sauce have significantly lower rates of prostate cancer. Other studies suggest lycopene can help prevent lung, colon and breast cancers. Tomatoes also contain the antioxidant glutathione, which helps boost immune function. Note: cooked tomatoes are preferable, since heat allows more antioxidants in tomatoes to be made available to the body. And because lycopene is fat-soluble, eating tomatoes with oil can improve absorption. (Subramanian 1987)

3. Red grapes – these are delicious frozen and served in lovely glasses for a cool summer dessert. I put a drop of rosewater-scented syrup on mine.

4. Garlic – perhaps the world's oldest known medicinal and culinary herb, is packed with antioxidants that can help fend off cancer, heart disease and the effects of aging. The sulfur compounds that give garlic its pungent odor are thought to be responsible for its healing benefits. Studies have shown that garlic keeps the heart healthy by low-

ering cholesterol levels, reducing blood pressure, fighting free radicals and keeping blood from clotting. Other studies suggest that eating garlic regularly can help prevent cancer. It also has potent anti-fungal properties and can help treat asthma and yeast infections.

6. Carrots – Carrots are loaded with a potent antioxidant called beta-carotene, a member of the healing family of carotenoids. Also found in beets, sweet potatoes and other yellow-orange vegetables, beta-carotene provides protection against cancer, especially lung, bladder, breast, esophageal and stomach cancers; heart disease, and the progression of arthritis by as much as 70 percent. Note: Lightly steamed carrots have considerably higher levels of antioxidants than uncooked, as the heat breaks down the active compounds and makes them more available. (Subramanian 1987)

7. Kale – this superfood is good for you in so many ways. I grind it up and hide it in foods and my kids eat a lot of it this way.

A recipe for bone stock:

Homemade stock enhances the flavor meat or vegetable soups, sauces and gravies. Any meat, poultry or fish can be used. Vegetables can be onions, garlic, celery or just about anything you have laying around that you need to get rid of. Greens are also good. All vegetables should be rough cut. (This is great stuff to help recover from hemolysis, as is liver and grape juice, too.)

- Add meat (poultry or fish) to a hot pot with a bit of fat in the bottom to keep the meat from sticking. Cook on medium high, stirring occasionally until slightly brown. Add rough cut vegetables and continue to cook until vegetables are soft. Add enough water to cover about two inches.

- When water boils, turn the heat down to low and add a lid to the pot. Simmer until meat falls off the bones. About 1 ½ hours.

- Strain into a jar or bowl and put in the refrigerator. The fat can be removed easily after it cools because it will solidify on top of the stock.

Notes:

CHAPTER 10

Drugs to Avoid

CONTRAINDICATED DRUG	LEVEL OF RISK
Acetaminophen	Low Risk
Acetanilid	High Risk
Acetylphenylhydrazine	High Risk
Aminophenazone	Low Risk
Antazoline	Low Risk
Antipyrine	Low Risk
Ascorbic acid (Hallberg 1986)	Low Risk
Aspirin	High Risk
Astemizole	High Risk

CONTRAINDICATED DRUG	LEVEL OF RISK
Beta- Naphthol	High Risk
Chloramphenicol	High Risk
Chloroquine	High Risk
Ciprofloxacin	High Risk
Colchicine	Low Risk
Dapsone	High Risk
Dimercaprol	High Risk
Diphenhydramine	Low Risk
Dopamine	Low Risk
Doxorubicin	High Risk
Ethanol	High Risk
Furazolidone	High Risk
Furosemide	High Risk
Gadopentetate dimeglumine	High Risk
Glucosulfone	High Risk
Glyburide	High Risk
Henna	High Risk
Ibuprofen	Low Risk
Isobutyl Nitrite	High Risk

CONTRAINDICATED DRUG	LEVEL OF RISK
Isoniazid	Low Risk
Lamotrigine	High Risk
Levofloxacin	High Risk
Lisinopril	high Risk
Magnevist	High Risk
Mefloquine	High Risk
Menadiol Sodium Sulfate (Vitamin k4 sodium sulfate)	High Risk
Menadione	High Risk
Menadione sodium Bisulfite (Vitamin K3 sodium bisulfite)	High Risk
Menthol	High Risk
Mesalazine	High Risk
Metformin	High Risk
Methylene Blue	High Risk
Mirtazapine	Low Risk
Moxifloxacin	High Risk
Nalidixic Acid	High Risk
Naphthalene	High Risk
Nimesulide	High Risk
Niridazole	High Risk

CONTRAINDICATED DRUG	LEVEL OF RISK
Nitrofurantoin	High Risk
Nitrofurazone	High Risk
Norfloxacin	Low Risk
Oxidase, Urate	High Risk
Pamaquine	High Risk
Para- Aminobenzoic Acid	Low Risk
Pefloxacin	High Risk
Pentaquine	High Risk
Phenacetin	High Risk
Phenazopyridine	High Risk
Phenylbutazone	Low Risk
Phenylhydrazine	High Risk
Phenytoin	Low Risk
Primaquine	High Risk
Probenecid	High Risk
Procainamide	Low Risk
Proguanil	Low Risk
Pyrimethamine	Low Risk
Quinacrine	High Risk

CONTRAINDICATED DRUG	LEVEL OF RISK
Quinidine	Low Risk
Quinine	Low Risk
Stibophen	High Risk
Streptomycin	Low Risk
Sulfacetamide	High Risk
Sulfacytine	Low Risk
Sulfadiazine	Low Risk
Sulfadimidine	High Risk
Sulfafurazole	High Risk
Sulfaguanidine	Low Risk
Sulfamerazine	Low Risk
Sulfamethoxazole	High Risk
Sulfamethoxypyridazine	Low Risk
Sulfanilamide	High Risk
Sulfapyridine	High Risk
Sulfasalazine	High Risk
Sulfathiazole	High Risk
Sulfonylurea	Low Risk
Sulfoxone	High Risk

CONTRAINDICATED DRUG	LEVEL OF RISK
Tamsulosin	High Risk
Tiaprofenic Acid	Low Risk
Toluidine Blue	High Risk
Trihexyphenidyl	Low Risk
Trimethoprim	Low Risk
Trinitrotoluene	High Risk
Tripelennamine	Low Risk
Vitamin K1	Low Risk

CHAPTER 11

Foods to Avoid

In the past six years I have recieved numerous comments from people who struggled, or whose children have struggled, with varying degrees of hemolysis. I have always advised them to try staying away from ALL legumes, as I have found that all legumes can cause oxidative stress (not just fava beans). I cannot count the letters of appreciation that I have gotten. I receive letters, almost weekly, from very grateful moms who finally have seen a huge difference in their child's health...just from diligently avoiding legumes, as well as the other items on this list of foods to avoid. This list of foods and substances to avoid names every legume I could find. Because even chronic low level hemolysis is very hard to detect, and can cause other health problems, I strongly recommend the avoidance of ALL legumes.

Here is a list of the foods and substances which are known to be possible triggers for hemolysis in people with G6PD deficiency:

Sulfites

• Sulfites are used in a wide variety of foods, so be sure to check labels carefully. (See Chapter 9: "Diet Suggestions" for more information on sufites)

Menthol

• Menthol can be difficult to avoid as tooth paste, candy, breath mints, mouth wash and many other products have menthol added to them. Mint from natural mint oils is alright to consume.

Artificial blue food coloring

• Other artificial food colors can also cause hemolysis. Natural food colors, such as found in foods like turmeric or grapes, are okay.

Ascorbic acid and iron

• Artificial ascorbic acid commonly put in food and vitamins can cause hemolysis in large doses and should be avoided. It is put into so many foods that you can be getting a lot of ascorbic acid without realizing it as is added to many prepared foods. Manufacturers make no distinction on their food labels between natural Vitamin C (citric acid) and ascorbic acid

Iron supplements

• Iron is released into the blood stream during hemolysis. It can even be fatal if the levels are high enough. There is evidence that ascorbic acid increases the body's ability to absorption of iron. (Lei 2008) Because of the problems of hemolysis in people with G6PDD, it is not uncommon for their levels to be abnormally high. This increased absorption could bring their iron to unhealthy levels. Consequently, NEVER give iron supplements to a G6PDD person without testing iron levels. It should only be done given under a Doctor's (who understands the problem) supervision. G6PDD people should have their iron levels tested regularly as iron overload can cause heart and liver problems.

Vitamin K

- Vitamin K^3 (Menadione) injections were standard procedure for newborns years ago to help prevent internal bleeding. However, it was found to cause hemolysis and it has been replaced by Vitamin K^1 (Phylloquinone) injections. However, Vitamin K injections as standard procedure for newborns is still controversial because there are still known risks associated with its use. Many doctors are proposing that Vitamin K injections at birth be used on a case by case basis. Even though the most recent reports say the risks are minimal, we recommend that moms opt out unless your baby is at very high risk of internal bleeding due to a deficiency of Vitamin K. There are other ways to make sure your baby has enough Vitamin K before he or she is born, as it is contraindicated in large doses, even for adults. (For more information read Chapter 4: "Caring for Babies with G6PD Deficiency")

Tonic water

- Tonic water contains quinine, a contraindicated drug which causes hemolysis in G6PDD people

Bitter gourd and garden egg

- Bitter Gourd is also known as Bitter Mellon. These are common foods in some parts of Africa and Asia.

Some Chinese herbs

- Particularly Rhizoma Coptidis (huang lien), Calculus Bovis (neu huang), Flos Chimonanthi Praecocis (leh mei hua), Flos Lonicerae (kam ngan fa) and Margarita or anything containing them.

BEANS

- Aduki bean
- adzuki bean
- azuki bean
- anasazi beans
- appaloosa bean
- asuki bean
- azufrado bean
- azuki bean
- baby lima bean
- bayo bean
- bengal bean
- black azuki bean
- black bean
- black turtle bean
- bolita bean
- bonavist bean
- borlotti bean
- Boston bean
- Boston navy bean
- broad bean
- brown speckled cow bean
- buffalo bean
- butter bean
- butterscotch calypso bean
- calypso bean
- canaria bean
- canario bean
- cannellini bean
- chestnut lima bean
- chili bean
- Christmas lima bean
- cabeca-de-frade
- chiporro
- coco bean-French white bean
- coco blanc bean-French white bean

BEANS (CONT.)

- crab eye bean
- Couhage
- Cowage
- Cowhage
- Cowitch
- cranberry bean
- dermason bean
- Dolichos pruriens
- edamame
- Egyptian bean
- Egyptian white broad bean
- English bean
- European soldier bean
- eye of the goat bean
- faba
- fagiolo romano
- fava bean
- fava-coceira
- fayot

- fazolia bean
- feijao bean
- feve
- field pea
- flageolet
- fool
- foul
- frijo bola roja
- frijole negro
- Fuji mame
- ful
- great Northern bean
- green gram
- haba
- habas
- haricot blanc bean
- horse bean
- hyacinth bean
- itchy bean

BEANS (CONT.)

- Indian bean
- Jackson wonder bean
- Jacob's cattle bean
- krame
- kidney bean
- lablab bean
- lima bean
- lingot bean
- lupini bean
- Madagascar bean
- maicoba bean
- maine Yellow eye
- mayocoba bean
- marrow bean
- mauritius bean
- Mexican black bean
- Mexican red bean
- molasses face bean
- mortgage lifter bean

- mortgage runner bean
- moth dal
- mucuna bean
- mucuna pruriens
- mucuna prurita
- mung bean
- mung pea
- mungo bean
- navy bean
- nescafe
- orca bean
- pea bean
- pearl haricot
- Peruano bean
- Peruvian bean
- picapica
- pink bean
- pinto bean
- po de mico

BEANS (CONT.)

- prince bean
- purple appaloosa bean
- rajma
- rattlesnake bean
- red ball bean
- red bean
- red eye bean
- red chori
- red kidney bean
- red Oriental bean
- rice bean
- rosecoco bean
- roman bean
- runner bean
- saluggia
- salugia bean
- scarlet runner bean
- Setae Siliquae Hirsutae
- shell bean

- small red bean
- small white bean
- soy bean
- soya bean
- soybean
- Spanish black bean
- Spanish Tolosana bean
- speckled brown cow bean
- Steuben yellow bean
- Steuben yellow eye bean
- Stizolobium pruriens
- Sweet bean
- Swedish brown bean
- tapary bean
- tepary bean
- Tiensin red bean
- Tolosana bean
- tongues of fire bean
- tremmocos

BEANS (CONT.)

- trout bean
- turtle bean
- turtle soup bean
- vallarta bean
- val
- velvet bean
- wax bean
- white bean
- white kidney bean
- white pea bean

- Windsor bean
- Yankee bean
- yellow Indian woman bean
- yin yang bean

BEAN PRODUCTS

- black beans in salted sauce
- black salted fermented bean
- Chinese black bean
- dow see
- fermented black bean

- frijoles refritos
- refried beans
- salted black bean
- salty black bean

SNAP BEANS (NOT-DRIED)

- asparagus bean
- asparagus pea
- bodi
- boonchi
- chepil
- Chinese long bean
- dau gok
- dow gok
- dragon tongue bean
- French bean
- French green bean
- four-angled bean
- goa bean
- green bean
- haricot verts
- Italian flat bean
- long bean
- manila bean
- princess pea
- romano bean
- runner bean
- sator
- snap bean
- string bean
- Thailand long bean
- wax bean
- winged bean
- winged pea
- yard-long bean

EDIBLE POD

- Chinese pea pod
- Chinese pea
- Chinese snow pea
- edible-podded pea
- mange-tout pea
- snow pea
- sugar pea
- sugar snap

LENTILS

- arhar
- arhar dal
- beluga black lentil
- beluga lentil
- Bengal gram
- black beluga lentil
- black chickpeas
- black gram
- black lentil
- brown lentil
- channa dal
- chana dal
- chilke urad
- chowli dal
- continental lentil
- dal
- daal
- dhaal
- dhal
- dhall
- Egyptian lentil
- French green lentils
- German lentil
- gram dal

LENTILS (CONT.)

- green lentil
- horse gram
- Indian brown lentil
- kala channa
- kali dal
- lablab beans
- lentilles du Puy
- lentilles vertes du Puy
- masar
- masar dal
- masoor
- masoor dal
- matki
- moath
- moong dal

- mussoor
- mussoor dal
- petite beluga lentil
- Puy lentil
- red lentil
- toor
- toor dal
- tuvar
- tuvar dal
- tur
- tur dal
- urad dal
- val dal
- white lentil
- yellow lenti

PEAS

- Bengal gram
- black-eyed pea
- black-eye bean
- black-eye pea
- black-eyed suzy
- ceci bean
- cici bean
- China bean
- chawli
- chickpea
- chick-pea
- chole
- congo pea
- congo bean
- cowpea
- crowder pea
- dried peas
- Egyptian pea
- field peas
- fresh peas
- gandules
- garbanzo bean
- garbanzo pea
- garbonzo bean
- goongoo pea
- green pea
- green matar dal
- green split pea
- gunga pea
- gungo pea
- kabuli channa
- kabli chana
- kabli channa
- lobhia
- locust bean
- lombia
- no-eyed peas
- pigeon pea

PEAS (CONT.)

- pois chiches
- poor man's pea
- Southern pea
- white chickpea

- yellow pea
- yellow matar dal
- yellow-eyed pea

SOY PRODUCTS

- abura-age
- aburage
- aka miso
- akamiso
- atsu-age
- atsuage
- bamboo yuba
- barley miso
- awase miso
- bean cheese
- bean curd
- bean curd sheets
- bean curd skins
- bean curd stick
- bean paste
- bean sauce
- bean stick
- brown rice miso
- Chinese yuba

- dark miso
- deep fat fried tofu
- deep-fried tofu
- doufu
- dow fu kon
- dried bean curd stick
- dried bean stick
- extra-firm tofu
- fermented bean cake
- fermented bean curd
- fermented soy cheese
- firm tofu
- foo yu
- fried bean curd
- fu jook pei
- fu yi
- fu yu
- genmai miso
- hat-cho miso

SOY PRODUCTS (CONT.)

- hatcho miso
- inaka miso
- inariage
- kinu-goshi
- kirazu
- kyoto shiro miso
- mame miso
- mamemiso
- medium tofu
- mellow white miso
- miso
- mugi miso
- nama-age
- nama nori san
- nato
- natto
- nattou
- nigari tofu
- okara

- plant protein
- preserved bean curd
- pressed tofu
- protein crumbles
- red miso
- regular tofu
- roasted soybeans
- sendai miso
- shinshu miso
- shiro miso
- shiromiso
- silken tofu
- soft tofu
- soy cheese
- soy mayonnaise
- soy milk
- soy milk skins
- soy sour cream
- soy nuts

SOY PRODUCTS (CONT.)

- soy yogurt
- soya cheese
- soya mayonnaise
- soybean curd
- soybean paper
- soybean paste
- soynuts
- soy nut butter
- soynut butter
- sui-doufu
- sweet miso
- sweet white miso
- tempe
- tempeh
- textured soy protein
- texturized soy protein
- textured vegetable protein
- texturized vegetable protein
- tofu
- tofu mayonnaise
- tofu sour cream
- TSP
- TVP
- uba
- unohana
- usu-age
- usuage
- vegetable protein
- wet bean curd
- white miso
- yellow miso
- yuba

VEGITABLE GUM THICKENERS
These are either made from legumes, or can be made from legumes

- albumin - from peas
- Acacia gum
- carob bean gum
- Flavoring or natural flavoring
- gum arabic
- guar gum
- lecithin
- locust bean gum

- Monosodium Glutamate (from soy)
- Tara seed gum
- tragacanth
- Vegetable broth (soy or even fava beans)
- vegetable emulsifier
- vegetable glycerin
- Vegetable gelatin
- vegetable stabilizer

OTHER LEGUMES

- Other Legumes
- Alfalfa sprouts
- Astragalus (herbal medicine)
- Carob (chocolate substitute)
- Fenugreek
- Jicama
- Licorice
- Peanuts

- Rooibos
- Red Tea
- African Red Tea
- Senna or Cassia
- Singkamas
- Tamarind
- Vetch Family (Not normally used for food)

OTHER FOODS THAT ALMOST ALWAYS CONTAIN SOY) (OR OTHER LEGUMES) OR SOY PRODUCTS)

- Artificial butter flavor

- Baked goods

- Candies

- Canned meats or tuna

- Canned soups

- Chips

- Chinese food

- Gravy Mixes

- Infant formula

- Low fat cheeses or cheese substitutes

- Margarine

- Sausages, hot dogs, processed meats

- Sauces (Worcestshire. Sweet and Sour etc)

- Salad Dressings

- Stock or bouillon

- Tofutti

- Powdered foods

Notes:

CHAPTER 13

Comments and Stories by Others

I'll also say thanks again, the information you provide has been life saving and affirming. Since changing our daughter's diet almost 4 years ago, her life has changed so much, she is active and healthy. Recently when she was contemplating the possibility of being somewhere without her parents (we double check all ingredients - she checks then we check) she said – but I'd have to have THE LIST! What would her life be without the list?

Thanks, Stacy

Had a lot of joint pain, after I stopped eating the foods to avoid it has stopped, my workouts have changed it was getting hard to bench 225 after diet change go 4 reps, big change THANK YOU SO MUCH

My son has had terrible headaches for the last 6 yrs since he had a hemolytic crisis. We have cut out all the contraindicated foods (Drs told us only to avoid fava beans) for the last few months and since then he has had no headaches!! We also take NAC daily which helps a lot especially with my fatigue and his behaviour. Anna

----

I just wanted you to know that with your help in reducing oxidative stress through organic food, watching triggers, increasing antioxidant consumption and supplementation in antioxidants as well as specific chiropractic care my son has gone from averaging 8 rbc to a normal 12-13. He is now 15 plays baseball, basketball and runs around full of vitality. Thanks for your help and you have made a huge difference in a child's life. Way to go!! Dr. Dean

----

At the suggestion of what Dale teaches us at his website, I have been taking Pine Bark and Niacin(No flush), Vitamin B6, folic acid, etc. for the past two weeks; I am already sleeping better and having more energy. One thing I really notice is that my breathing is deeper and more relaxed. Well, I may or may not have G6PD deficiency, but these supplements may just give me a better life, and to my sister and her son(who is G6PD deficient) a new life. Thank you Dale for providing your help with your website. Sui.

----

dales book is the best. We live by it. The recipes r now all our favorites... dale is a blessing to us all. Get the book on his site.. Lynda

----

Thank you Dale. I can't express how much we are benefiting from all you can share with us. God Bless. Best regards, Maitha

----

I want to thank you again for creating this wonderful website, I feel it has solved a big mystery that I've had life long, since I have always felt unwell but never knew I had G6PD deficiency! Love and blessings, Rosina

----

I told you I would follow up with my son's healing progress. This past September, JT was showing signs of hemolysis so we took him to the hematolgist to have his blood checked (we hadn't been in 10 years). Thankfully his blood did not indicate hemolysis; however, he was slightly jaundice and his urine was the color of ice tea (Hematologist told us he was severely G6PDD - 0.7). When we were told JT was G6PDD as an infant, we were only give a short list of contraindicated items (i.e., sulfa, mothballs and fava beans). Since I bought your book and constantly browsing this website, we've removed as much as we are aware from JT's diet (as well as mine as I am G6PDD too) of the contraindicated items. That being said, his urine color has changed back to normal and his eyes are no longer yellow.

I praise Yahu my Elohim for the healing of JT's body, for wisdom, understanding and a peace of mind, and for you and for this website!

Our daughter is adopted. She has favism. It has made a big change in our life, particularly in what we eat, but changing her diet has made a huge change in her life - she is so much healthier and happier.

Our son is g6hp deficient so we have opted for the whole family to follow his diet.... After many hours reading about all the additives and junk put in almost all processed and some supposedly fresh foods. we have totally changed our diet as well. I firmly believe that almost all the things that our son Trevor can not have are also bad for everyone as well..Dare I say it, but I am starting to think this is a blessing more than anything as it has opened our eyes to a new way of living and eating.

We use baking soda instead of tooth paste like our great grandparents did. Also Mild soap for shampoo and olive oil, grape seed oil or best coconut oil make great hair conditioner. Our mosquito repellent is coconut oil and apple cider vinegar. Really there is no need for expensive products full of deadly toxins. In Philippines we can get fresh coco beans and make chocolate that is better than any shop brought stuff. We are learning to make treats and every day things that are healthy and really so inexpensive, the main cost is time but our family's health is worth it. We will be getting Dales book as soon as we can...

----

hi there. i'm a first time mother of 2 months old raijin and he has g6pd deficiency...and as a mother, i want to give my child all best care i have specially in taking foods and medicines...i'm very thankful i found your website who supports children with g6pd deficiency and now i'm very much more aware of his diet and as early as today i have more ideas on how to take care of my baby in the future....thanks a lot and god bless!

My son was finally diagnosed with G6PD when he was around 5 months after countless trips to GP and doctors all of which didn't listen. I knew as a mother of 3 my son being my 3rd that he was ill especially in a lot of pain when taking antibiotics but I was branded as a bad mother because I stopped giving them. He was missed diagnosed with thalassemia which he is only a trait the thalassemia society picked up that his condition was not the signs of a carrier and helped me find someone that I could consultant with in the society to help me. He is

8 years old now its been a fight all along. My current gp still is not sure how to treat him and most gps haven't heard of the condition. Teachers and teacher assistants constantly have to be reminded. A recent issue of which i picked up on was moth balls used by a teacher assistant made my son very ill and physical education is getting harder and harder with his breathing. God help him and me in secondary school. People have got to be more aware.

Hi sir. I just recently added the Support G6PD Awareness Cause to my facebook account. I currently work as a nurse in the Newborn Screening Center- Mindanao here in the Philippines and I deal with G6PD patients all the time. I would just like to say that I am glad that you have made this as a cause because this disorder is becoming more rampant, esp. here in the Philippines. take care and Keep that fire burning :) More power.

---

i am a neonatal ICU nurse your website is very much helpful for me, my son and my patients. thank you very much!

Hello all Many thanks to Dale, Dr O and all the good people who contribute to this group. It really has helped those parents who have kids with G6PD def, I remember my initial shock at being told my kid had the def- I panicked and had no clue what to do. All the Dr could say was since you live in a malaria prone area don't take any of d 'quines' sadly I guess that was all she knew. I started trying to get more information and thankfully I saw this group. Thank you all for the good work you do. I have been a member of this group for a while (albeit a quiet one as I am not much of a writer) my baby girl turns 2 in a few days and I am so thankful to GOD. GOD bless you.

I am one of those patients labeled hypochondriac, lazy and worse...I almost have to cry every time I need the doctor to check me or my son because of some infection that makes us feel just miserable, I didn't know about these chronic micro hemolysis, and the devastating effect they have on our entire body, with this information I now can at last talk to my son's school teachers about his chronic fatigue, and maybe convince my doctor to listen to me instead of dismissing me as a nutcase!!!

Thank you, thank you, thank you all, Dr. Ogundu, Dale and everybody else who share their knowledge with us.

I am happy to have found this site, and relieved to see that we are not alone in this; now, with all the information I already have found , and more I'm sure I will get in the future, I can try to explain to everybody around us that we are not lazy (at work or at school), and that we really need to rest a lot when we are feeling sick, and that we really get sick that often, it is not in our heads, it's real.

I finally can stand up straight and say: I am not faking, I am sick, not crazy!!!! thank you for the support

----

I know I did it before, but I'm going to thank Dale for this website, and dr. Orgundu for all the experience shared here with us... thanks to all that I had a great day: today I had a meeting at my son's school with the headmaster and the school healthcare coordinator (I hope you say it like this...), to explain about his condition, and for the first time I could explain it in such a manner that everybody understood why my son is sick and so tired all the time, they are looking at him in a different manner, with understanding not suspicion, and they are going to keep an eye on him, and try to help him as much as they can.... what a relief , I felt understood for the first time. I didn't have the same luck with my doctor, but I don't despair anymore, I know enough to keep us as healthy as possible, and next month we are going to a special doctor, an orthomolecular physician that will check our blood for just anything .

Dale, thanks for the food suggestions. My son is up and kicking again. I made the chicken stock and found pomegranate juice and I am feeding him only good food (lots of red meat as well) so THANK YOU for all the good advice.

whishing you all the best. (a very happy mother)

Hi thanks for the book, I really appreciate it! My 8 months old baby boy recently got diagnosed with G6PD and I was looking on the net for some info when I came across your site. First of all GREAT JOB!!!!! It's nice to know we are not alone and there is someone who is willing to take time out to educate people on this disorder. Many thanks.

Thank you very much for the consideration you give to our case. I really feel that just now I can fully understand my case after I entered your website. God bless you and the hard work you do to help us.

Totally agree with Dale. We should not just blindly follow doctor's order because in my son's case, it turns out he easily got sick and we didn't know why until we changed his diet....

The diet and the things people have discussed with supplements in this group has helped my son tremendously. Definitely let your doctor know about the symptoms and please do not accept "let's wait and see".

Since I discovered your site, I have been cautious with what we eat, reading all the labels, and I must say, I feel better, I have more energy, don't feel like a 90 years old anymore...maybe this can help those who aren't sure how important it is to follow a diet, it's worth trying, at the end you learn to eat healthy!

Ok, my son will be 1 yr in October, he was tested to be positive to g6pd at birth, and he had blood transfusion before we were discharged and we were told to avoid certain foods and drugs. But am so lucky to have met a doctor who told me that the list I was given will not give me the full info I needed and referred me to the web. I googled and found this site where so many people have been helpful on daily basis. My son is ok, no reaction to anything cos I am praying hard and as well trying hard to avoid any trigger.

If I hadn't found this group probably my son who is now 3 yrs old would have been sick always. When I tried to avoid all the triggers and contraindicated medicines, He became more healthy and active.

We are really the caretakers of our children and we should do what will be the best for them.

Thanks to the Group here especially to Dale who unselfishly feed us with knowledge to properly handle our health situation and make our precious child healthy as ever.

Having found this website is the best thing you could have done. Unfortunately for us and our children the doctors seem to/want to play down our condition to a point where we parents seem to flounder for some clear direction. You should spend time and read through this entire website and try and follow dietary restrictions and the medicine contra list as far as possible. Dale and many other contributors to this site have lived with this condition and are always ready to help us parents/patients. Do not hesitate to ask any questions you may have as you will probably/definitely get a response from someone somewhere around the globe. You will as I did realize that you are not alone in dealing with this condition.

Thanks for the support, now my wife is calming down after i give her an explanation that our baby can be grow normally and healthy.. God Bless You all..

Appendix

Glossary

anemia	A condition marked by a deficiency of red blood cells or of hemoglobin in the blood.
asymptomatic	Exhibiting or producing no symptoms.
bilirubin	A yellow protein that appears in the urine following the breakdown of hemoglobin.
chromosome	A structure in the nucleus containing a linear thread of DNA which transmits genetic information.
CNSHA	Congenital Non-Spherocytic Hemolytic Anemia (anemia caused by the loss of red blood cells that have been damaged due to an inherited trait)
contraindicate	To report the presence of a disease or physical condition that makes it impossible or undesirable to treat a particular client in the usual manner or to prescribe medicines that might otherwise be suitable.
enzyme	A protein that enables reactions between substances.
free radicals	An atom or group of atoms with at least one unpaired electron. In the body it is usually an oxygen molecule that has lost an electron and will stabilize itself by stealing an electron from a nearby molecule that results in damaging other cells
genetic	Pertaining to or produced by a gene; inherited.
glutathione	A polypeptide that is important in cellular respiration. It is a major protective mechanism against oxidative stress. It protects red blood cells from hydrogen peroxide, a toxic byproduct of certain metabolic reactions.

Glossary (continued)	
hemaglobin	A red protein responsible for transporting oxygen in the blood.
hemolysis	The break down of red blood cells.
hemolytic anemia	Anemia caused by the depletion of red blood cells.
jaundice	Yellow discoloration of the skin, the white of the eye, and other tissues caused by excessive bilirubin in the blood.
kernicterus	Brain deposition of bilirubin in neonate (newborns).
legumes	Legumes are plants in the pea family that produce pods that split open naturally along a seam, revealing a neat row of seeds.
Lyonization	The process by which all X chromosomes of the cells in excess of one are inactivated on a random basis.
parasites	An animal or plant that lives in or on another (the host) from which it obtains nourishment. The host does not benefit from the association and is often harmed by it.
petrochemicals	A chemical derived from petroleum or natural gas.
RBCs	Red blood cells
triggers	A factor that initiates and aggravates a situation.
Some of these definitions were used from the following online sources: http://www.angelfire.com/wv/MT/ http://medical-dictionary.thefreedictionary.com/ http://www.wisegeek.org/what-are-legumes.htm thefreedictionary.com	

Bibliography

Al-Omran, Abbas, MD, Fouad Al-Ghaz, MD, Samir Gupta, and Thomas B. John, MD. "GLUCOSE-6-PHOSPHATE DE-HYDROGENASE DEFICIENCY AND NEONATAL JAUNDICE IN AL-HOFUF AREA." Annals of Saudi Medicine, 19.2 (1999): 156+. National Center for Biotechnology Information. U.S. National Library of Medicine. Web. 19 Apr. 2013. <http://www.kfshrc.edu.sa/annals/Old/192/98-140.pdf>.

Alderson, Andrew. "Holy Straight Bananas – Now the Eurocrats Are Banning Moth Balls." Http://www.telegraph.co.uk/. The Telegraph, 18 Nov. 2008. Web. 18 Apr. 2013. <http://www.telegraph.co.uk/news/newstopics/howaboutthat/3463893/Holy-straight-bananas-now-the-Eurocrats-are-banning-moth-balls.html>.

Batetta, B., R. R. Bonatesta, F. Sanna, M. Putzolu, M. F. Mulas, M. Collu, and S. Dessì. "Cell growth and cholesterol metabolism in human glucose- 6-phosphate dehydrogenase deficient lymphomononuclear cells." BioInfoBank Library. June 2002. BioInfoBank Library. 10 Apr. 2013 <http://lib.bioinfo.pl/pmid:12027950>

Becana, M., and R. V. Klucas. "Transition metals in legume root nodules: Iron-dependent free radical production increases during nodule senescence." National Center for Biotechnology Information. 1 Oct. 1992. U.S. National Library of Medicine. 11 Apr. 2013. <http://www.ncbi.nlm.nih.gov/pmc/articles/PMC50043/>.

Beutler, Ernest, Mary Yeh, and Virgil F. Fairbanks. "THE NORMAL HUMAN FEMALE AS A MOSAIC OF X-CHROMO-SOME ACTIVITY: STUDIES USING THE GENE FOR G-6-PD-DEFICIENCY AS A MARKER." Proceedings of the

National Acadamy of Science U S A PMC285481 48 (1962). Proceedings of the National Acadamy of Science U S A. Jan. 1962. Proceedings of the National Acadamy of Science U S A. 11 Apr. 2013. < http://www.ncbi.nlm.nih.gov/pmc/articles/PMC285481/>.

Bhalla, Ashish, U. N. Jajoo, A. P. Jain, and S. P. Kalantri. "HAEMO-LYSIS WITH ANTI-MALARIAL DRUGS IN GLUCOSE 6 PHOSPHATE DEHYDROGENASE DEFICIENCY." Journal of Ayub Medical College, Abbottabad. 2004. Journal of Ayub Medical College, Abbottabad. 10 Apr. 2013. <http://www.ayubmed.edu.pk/JAMC/PAST/16-3/AshishBhalla.htm>.

Bocchetta, Alberto. "Psychotic mania in glucose-6-phosphate-dehydro-genase-deficient subjects." National Center for Biotechnology Information. 13 June 2003. U.S. National Library of Medicine. 11 Apr. 2013. < ww.ncbi.nlm.nih.gov/pmc/articles/PMC165592/>.

Büyükokuroğlu, Mehmet Emin, Sayit Altikat, and Mehmet Çiftçi. "The Effects of Ethanol on Glucose 6-phosphate Dehydro-genase Enzyme Activity from Human Erythrocytes in Vitro and Rat Erythrocytes in Vivo." 13 Feb. 2002. Oxford Journals. 10 Apr. 2013. <http://alcalc.oxfordjournals.org/content/37/4/327.full>.

Carson, P. E., C. L. Flanagan, C. E. Ickes, and A. S. Alving. "Enzymatic Deficiency in Primaquine-Sensitive Erythrocytes." Science 124 (1956): 484-85. National Center for Biotechnology Information. U.S. National Library of Medicine. 11 Apr. 2013. <http://www.sciencemag.org/content/124/3220/484.2.full.pdf?ijkey=5155f932d3a44c49027cc9415d0d2f7368ec8499&keytype2=tf_ipsecsha>.

Chan, T. K. "Glucose-6-Phosphate Dehydrogenase (G6PD) Deficiency: A Review." Glucose-6-Phosphate Dehydrogenase (G6PD) Deficiency: A Review. The University of Hong Kong. 10 Apr. 2013. <http://www.cchi.com.hk/specialtopic/case1/case1. htm>.

Devi, A. M. Shanthala, Rose Helen, Alwar Vanamala, and V. Chaithra. "Screening for G6PD Deficiency in Blood Donor Population." Editorial. Http://www.ncbi.nlm.nih.gov/. U.S. National Library of Medicine, 19 Oct. 2010. Web. Sept. 2010. <http:// www.ncbi.nlm.nih.gov/pmc/articles/PMC3002082/>.

Dhillon, A. S., P. J. Darbyshire, M. D. Williams,, and J. G. Bissenden. CASE REPORT Massive acute haemolysis in neonates with glucose-6- phosphate dehydrogenase deficiency. Rep. Disease in Childhood, 2002. <http://www.ncbi.nlm.nih.gov/pmc/articles/PMC1763238/pdf/v088p0F534.pdf>.

Elyassi, Cpt Ali R., and Maj Henry H. Rowshan. "Perioperative Management of the Glucose-6-Phosphate Dehydrogenase Deficient Patient: A Review of Literature." Anesthesia Progress Online. Anesthesia Progress, 14 Apr. 2009. Web. 10 Apr. 2013. < http://www.ncbi.nlm.nih.gov/pmc/articles/PMC2749581/>

Fiorelli, G., Martinez Di Montemuros, F, and Cappellini, MD. "Result Filters." Diss. University of Milan, 2000. Abstract. Chronic Non-spherocytic Haemolytic Disorders Associated with Glucose-6-phosphate Dehydrogenase Variants. U.S. National Library of Medicine, 13 Mar. 2000. Web. 19 Apr. 2013. <http:// www.ncbi.nlm.nih.gov/pubmed/10916677>.

Frank, Jennifer E. "Diagnosis and Management of G6PD Deficiency." Diagnosis and Management of G6PD Deficiency – October 1, 2005 – American Family Physician. 1 Oct. 2005. American Family Physician. 11 Apr. 2013 <http://www.aafp.org/afp/2005/1001/p1277.html>.

Fulghesu, Anna M., Francesca Sanna, Sabrina Uda, Roberta Magnini, Elaine Portoghese, and Barbara Batetta. "Production of Inflammatory Molecules in Peripheral Blood Mono-nuclear Cells from Severely Glucose-6-Phosphate Dehydrogenase-Deficient Subjects." National Center for Biotechnology Information. 20 Mar. 2011. U.S. National Library of Medicine. 10 Apr. 2013. <http://www.ncbi.nlm.nih.gov/pubmed/17361089>.

"G6PD." IHTC G6PD Comments. Indiana Hemophilia & Thrombosis Center, n.d. Web. 19 Apr. 2013. <http://www.ihtc.org/patient/blood-disorders/other-hematological-disorders/g6pd>.

"G6PD Deficiency Protects against Severe Malaria." Malaria. Public Library of Science, 7 Mar. 2013. Web. 19 Apr. 2013. <http://malaria.wellcome.ac.uk/doc_WTX037260.html>.

Gaskin, RS, D. Estwick, and R. Peddi. "G6PD deficiency: Its role in the high prevalence of hypertension and diabetes mellitus." National Center for Biotechnology Information. 2001. Geriatrics Hospital, St. Michael, Barbados, West Indies. 10 Apr. 2013. <http://www.ncbi.nlm.nih.gov/pubmed/11763298>.

"Glucose-6-Phosphate Dehydrogenase Deficiency." The Free Dictionary by Farlex. The Free Dictionary by Farlex, n.d. Web. 19 Apr. 2013. <http://medical-dictionary.thefreedictionary.com/G6PD+deficiency+anaemia>. Hallberg, L., M. Brune, and L. Rossander. "Effect of ascorbic acid on iron absorption from different types of meals. Studies with ascorbic-acid-rich foods and synthetic ascorbic acid given in different amounts with different meals." National Center for Biotechnology Information. Apr. 1986. U.S. National Library of Medicine. 10 Apr. 2013. <http://www.ncbi.nlm.nih.gov/pubmed/3700141>.

Halvorsen, Bente L.,Kari Holte, Mari C. W. Myhrstad, Ingrid Barikmo, Erlend Hvattum, Siv Fagertun Remberg, Anne-Brit Wold, Karin Haffner, Halvard Baugerød, Lene Frost Andersen, Ø. Moskaug, David R. Jacobs, Jr., and Rune Blomhoff. "A Systematic Screening of Total Antioxidants in Dietary Plants" J. Nutr. 2002 132: 3 461-471. < http://jn.nutrition.org/content/132/3/461.full.pdf+html>

J. Nutr. 2002 132: 3 461-471 Herschel, Marguerite, MD, Matthew Ryan, MD, Terri Gelbart, BS, and Michael Kaplan, MB, ChB. "Hemolysis and Hyperbilirubinemia in an African American Neonate Heterozygous for Glucose-6-Phosphate Dehydrogenase Deficiency." Nature.com. Nature Publishing Group, Oct. 2002. Web. 18 Apr. 2013. <http://nature.com/jp/journal/v22/n7/full/7210769a.html>.

Hershko, Chaim, and Robert S. Hillman. "Free Medical Textbook." Free Medical Textbook. 30 Dec. 2011. Medtextfee. 16 Apr. 2013. <http://medtextfree.wordpress.com/2011/12/30/chapter-59-acute-blood-loss-anemia/>.

Heymann, Anthony D., Yossi Cohen MD, and Gabriel Chodick PHD, MHA. "Glucose-6-Phosphate Dehydrogenase Deficiency and Type 2 Diabetes." Glucose-6-Phosphate Dehydrogenase Deficiency and Type 2 Diabetes. Aug. 2012. American Diabetes Association. 10 Apr. 2013. <http://care.diabetesjournals.org/content/35/8/e58.full>.

Huh, S. Y., Rifas-Shiman, S. L., Taveras, E. M., Oken, E., & Gillman, M. W. (2011). Timing of Solid Food Introduction and Risk of Obesity in Preschool-Aged Children. Pediatrics. doi:10.1542/peds.2010-0740 Web.16 Apr. 2013. < http://www.ncbi.nlm.nih.gov/pmc/articles/PMC3065143/>.

Ho, H.Y., , Cheng ML, Chiu DT. Glucose-6-phosphate Dehydrogenase – from Oxidative Stress to Cellular Functions and Degenerative Diseases. Diss. 2007. Philidelphia: Maney, 2007. Ingentaconnect.com. Maney Publlishing, June 2007. Web. 19 Apr. 2013. <http://www.ingentaconnect.com/content/

maney/rer/2007/00000012/00000003/art00001>.

Hussain, Mohammad, Mohammade Irshad, Musa Kalim, Liquat Ali, and Liaquat Ali. "GLUCOSE-6-PHOSPHATE DEHY-DROGENASE DEFICIENCY IN JAUNDICED NEO-NATES." JPM I 24.2 (2010): 122-26. Docs.google. Department of Pediatrics. Web. 19 Apr. 2013. <https://docs.google.com/viewer?a=v&q=cache:Mf77jYguVc8J:www.jpmi.org.pk/index.php/jpmi/article/download/1049/958+&hl=en&gl=us&pid=bl&srcid=ADGEESitfRjdXFX4DsOYeO3vmh-qYAWY-2Bocy4xpStLcYdfziqCp7UbYuGm7GAKCyg7Wb-7muPz833IG9m17d1uL0Q5RaFPaWqar0p-dXbkWsRgF-2DTHckMqK9QODBsABQvIgkddkWGoF&sig=AHI-EtbSKFiA8qq1UgOfiPRCLeDmPyTMICA>.

IGLESSIAS, J, Marli Auxiliadora C. et al. Erythrocyte glucose-6-phosphate dehydrogenase deficiency in male newborn babies and its relationship with neonatal jaundice. Rev. Bras. Hematol. Hemoter. [online]. 2010, vol.32, n.6 [cited 2013-04-19], pp. 434-438 . Available from: <http://www.scielo.br/scielo.php?script=sci_arttext&pid=S1516-84842010000600005&lng=en&nrm=i-so>. Epub July 30, 2010. ISSN 1516-8484. <http://dx.doi.org/10.1590/S1516-84842010005000086

"Jaundice and Kernicterus Symptoms, Causes, and Treatments on MedicineNet.com." MedicineNet. MedicineNet. 11 Apr. 2013. <http://www.medicinenet.com/kernicterus/article.htm>.

"Jaundice, Newborn." JPM I 24.2 (2010): 122-26. Jaundice, Newborn. 6 Feb. 2012. Web. 19 Apr. 2013. <http://www.nhs.uk/conditions/Jaundice-newborn/Pages/Introduction.aspx>.

Johnston, C. S., C. G. Meyer, and J. C. Srilakshmi. "Vitamin C elevates red blood cell glutathione in healthy adults." National Center for Biotechnology Information. July 1993. U.S. National Library of Medicine. 11 Apr. 2013. <http://ajcn.nutri-tion.org/content/58/1/103.full.pdf+html>.

"Kernicterus: MedlinePlus Medical Encyclopedia." U.S National Library of Medicine. U.S. National Library of Medicine. 11 Apr. 2013. <http://www.nlm.nih.gov/medlineplus/ency/article/007309.htm>.

Lei, J., M. Q. Zhang, C. Y. Huang, L. Bai, and Z. H. He. "Effects of Ascorbic Acid and Citric Acid on Iron Bioavailability in an in Vitro Digestion/ Caco-2 Cell Culture Model." National Center for Biotechnology Information. U.S. National Library of Medicine, 28 Oct. 2008. Web. 23 Apr. 2013. <http://www.ncbi.nlm.nih.gov/pubmed/18971162>.

Macknin ML, Medendorp SV, Maier MC. Infant sleep and bedtime cereal. Am J Dis Child. 1989 Sep;143(9):1066-8. PubMed PMID: 2672785. 15 Apr. 2013. <http://www.ncbi.nlm.nih.gov/pubmed/2672785>.

Marshall A. Lightman. National Academy of Science Ernest Beutler Biographical Memoir. Washington, D.C.: Marshall A. Lightman, 2012. Nasonline.org. National Academy of Science, 2012. Web. 18 Apr. 2013. <http://www.nasonline.org/publications/biographical-memoirs/memoir-pdfs/beutler-ernest.pdf>.

McKusick, Victor A., Alan F. Scott, Moyra Smith, Michael J. Wright, Ada Hamosh, Deborah L. Stone, Marla J. F. O'Neill, and Cassandra L. Kniffin. "GLUCOSE-6-PHOSPHATE DE-HYDROGENASE; G6PD." GLUCOSE-6-PHOSPHATE DEHYDROGENASE; G6PD. 6 July 1987. OMIM. 11 Apr. 2013. <http://omim.org/entry/305900>.

"Misdiagnosis of Anemia." - RightDiagnosis.com. Right Diagno-

sis from Health Grades, 1 Mar. 2013. Web. 19 Apr. 2013.
<http://www.rightdiagnosis.com/a/anemia/misdiag.htm>.

Moiz, Bushra, Amna Nasir, Sarosh Ahmed Khan, Salima Amin Kher-
ani, and Maqbool Qadir. "Abstract." National Center for Biotechnology Information. U.S. National Library of Medicine,
20 Aug. 2012. Web. 19 Apr. 2013. <http://www.ncbi.nlm.
nih.gov/pmc/articles/PMC3529675/>.

Muntoni, S. "Gene-Nutrient Interactions in G6PD-Deficient Subjects – Implications for Cardiovascular Disease Susceptibility." Gene-Nutrient Interactions in G6PD-Deficient Subjects
– Implications for Cardiovascular Disease Susceptibility. Oct.
2007. Journal of Nutrigenet and Nutrigenomics. 10 Apr.
2013. <http://www.karger.com/Article/FullText/109874>.

Nicol, Christopher J., Julian Zielenski, Lap-Chee Tsui, and Peter G.
Wells. An embryoprotective role for glucose-6-phosphate dehydrogenase in developmental oxidative stress and chemical
teratogenesis. Rep. 1st ed. Vol. 14. 111-127. FASEB J, 2000.
An embryoprotective role for glucose-6-phosphate dehydrogenase in developmental oxidative stress and chemical teratogenesis. Jan. 2000. FASEB J. 10 Apr. 2013. <http://care.
diabetesjournals.org/content/35/8/e58.full>.

Reclos, George J., Christine J. Hatzidakis, Eurico Camargo Neto,
Claudio Sampaio Jr, and Kenneth A. Pass. "A NEW RAPID
ASSAY USING OUR "HEMOGLOBIN NORMALIZA-
TION" METHOD FOR THE DETERMINATION OF
G-6-PD ACTIVITY IN NEONATES." R & D Diagnostics,
Ltd. R & D Diagnostics, Ltd. 10 Apr. 2013. < http://www.
rddiagnostics.com/article7.htm>.

Reclos, G. J., C. J. Hatzidakis, and K. H. Schulpis. "Glucose-6-Phos-
phate Dehydrogenase Neonatal Screening : Preliminary evi-

dence that a high percentage of partially deficient female neonates is missed during routine screening." National Center for Biotechnology Information. 1 Mar. 2000. U.S. National Library of Medicine. 10 Apr. 2013. <http://www.ncbi.nlm.nih.gov/pubmed/10807147>.

Rees, D. C., H. Kelsey, and J. D. Richards. "Acute haemolysis induced by high dose ascorbic acid in glucose-6-phosphate dehydrogenase deficiency." US National Library of Medicine. 27 Mar. 1993. PubMed. 15 Apr. 2013. <http://www.ncbi.nlm.nih.gov/pmc/articles/PMC1677333/>.

Rothville, Karin, DipCBEd. "Vitamin K: A Literature Review By Karin Rothville DipCBEd." Vitamin K: A Literature Review By Karin Rothville DipCBEd. Karin Rothville, 17 Feb. 2011. Web. 10 Apr. 2013. < http://www.whale.to/a/rothville.html>

Seidlein, Lorenz von, Sarah Auburn, Fe Espino, Dennis Shanks, Qin Cheng, James McCarthy, Kevin Baird, Catherine Moyes, Rosalind Howes, Didier Ménard, Germana Bancone, Ari Winasti-Satyahraha, Lasse S Vestergaard, Justin Green, Gonzalo Domingo, Shunmay Yeung, Ric Price Malar J. "Review of key knowledge gaps in glucose-6-phosphate dehydrogenase deficiency detection with regard to the safe clinical deployment of 8-aminoquinoline treatment regimens: a workshop report." 2013; 12: 112. Published online 2013 March 27. doi: 10.1186/1475-2875-12-112. <http://www.ncbi.nlm.nih.gov/pmc/articles/PMC3616837/citedby/?forwardCitationCount=0&citedOnBiomedCentral=false7>

Silliman, Christopher C., Lynn K. Boshkov, Zahra Mehdizadehkashi, David J. Elzi, William O. Dickey, Linda Podlosky, Gwen Clarke, and Daniel R. Ambruso. "Transfusion-related acute lung injury: Epidemiology and a prospective analysis of etiologic factors." Transfusion-related acute lung injury: Epidemiology and a prospective analysis of etiologic factors. 5 Sept. 2002. Journal of the American Society of Hematology. 10

Apr. 2013. <http://bloodjournal.hematologylibrary.org/content/101/2/454.full>.

Staff, Mayo Clinic. "Anemia." Mayo Clinic. 08 Mar. 2013. Mayo Foundation for Medical Education and Research. 10 Apr. 2013. <http://www.mayoclinic.com/health/anemia/DS00321/DSECTION=symptoms>.

Stanton, Robert C., M.D. "Robert C. Stanton, M.D. Research Summary." Stanton, Robert C., M.D. Joslin Diabetes Center, n.d. Web. 10 Apr. 2013. Article link

Subramanian, Shashma. "Fact or Fiction: Raw veggies are healthier than cooked ones: Scientific American." Fact or Fiction: Raw veggies are healthier than cooked ones: Scientific American. 31 Mar. 2009. 16 Apr. 2013. <https://store.joslin.org/diabetes-research/Robert-Stanton-MD.html>.Sklar, G. E. "Hemolysis as a Potential Complication of Acetaminophen Overdose in a Patient With Glucose-6-Phosphate Dehydrogenase Deficiency." National Center for Biotechnology Information. May 2002. U.S. National Library of Medicine. 10 Apr. 2013 <http://www.medscape.com/viewarticle/434465_3>

Sultana, Nayma, Noorzahan Begum, Shelina Begum, Sultana Ferdousi, and Taskina Ali. "Effects of vitamin E supplementation on some aspects of hematological variables in patients of hemolytic anemia with glucose 6 phosphate dehydrogenase (G6PD) deficiency." Effects of vitamin E supplementation on some aspects of hematological variables in patients of hemolytic anemia with glucose 6 phosphate dehydrogenase (G6PD) deficiency. 2006. Bangladesh Journal of Physiology and Pharmacology. 10 Apr. 2013. < http://www.banglajol.info/index.php/BJPP/article/viewArticle/3563>.

Tarnow-Mordi, William O., Nick J. Evans, Kei Lui, and Brian Darlow. "Risk of Brain Damage in Babies from Naphthalene in

Mothballs: Call to Consider a National Ban." Medical Journal of Australia. Committe of the Austrailian and New Zealand Neonatal Network, Aug. 2011. Web. 18 Apr. 2013. <https://www.mja.com.au/journal/2011/194/3/risk-brain-damage-babies-naphthalene-mothballs-call-consider-national-ban>.

United States of America. Department of the Army. Third US Army US Army Forces Central LCC. Malaria Journal. By AFRDSURG. Third U.S. Army/USARCENT/CFLCC, 2006. Web. 20 Apr. 2013. <http://www.malariajournal.com/content/12/1/112>.

Valiaveedan, Sebastian, Charu Mahajan, Girija P. Rath, Ashish Bindra, and Manish K. Marda. "Possible fenugreek induced haemolysis in a patient with previously unknown G6PD deficiency." National Center for Biotechnology Information. 01 July 0005. U.S. National Library of Medicine. 10 Apr. 2013. <http://www.ncbi.nlm.nih.gov/.pmc/articles/PMC3057251/>.

"VITAMIN K1 (phytonadione) Injection, Emulsion [Hospira, Inc.]." RSS. Daily Med, Apr. 2011. Web. 18 Apr. 2013. <http://dailymed.nlm.nih.gov/dailymed/lookup.cfm?setid=e8808230-2c44-44c6-8cab-8f29b6b34051>.

"Vitamins: Search Results." For the University of Maryland Medical Center Website. University of Maryland Medical Center, n.d. Web. 20 Apr. 2013. <http://www.umm.edu/search-results.htm?q=vitamins>.

Washington, E. C., W. Ector, M. Abboud, B. Ohning, and K. Holden. "Hemolytic jaundice due to G6PD deficiency causing kernicterus in a female newborn." National Center for Biotechnology Information. July 1995. U.S. National Library of Medicine. 11 Apr. 2013. <http://www.ncbi.nlm.nih.gov/pubmed/7597488>.

"Which Vitamins are Antioxidants." Http://thistimethisspace.com/. This Time This Space, 10 March 2013. Web. 20 Apr. 2013. <http://thistimethisspace.com/2010/03/19/which-vitamins-are-antioxidants/>.

Wright, R. O., H. E. Perry, A. D. Woolf, and M. W. Shannon. "Hemolysis after acetaminophen overdose in a patient with glucose-6-phosphate dehydrogenase deficiency." National Center for Biotechnology Information. 1996. U.S. National Library of Medicine. 10 Apr. 2013. <http://informahealthcare.com/doi/abs/10.3109/15563659609013837>.

"X-chromosome inactivation." Genetics Home Reference. Genetics Home Reference. 11 Apr. 2013. <http://ghr.nlm.nih.gov/glossary=xchromosomeinactivation>

Zhang, Zhaoyun, Chong Wee Liew, Diane E. Hardy, Yingyi Zhang, Jane A. Leopold, Ji Hi, Lili Guo, Rohit N. Kulkami, Joseph Loscalzo, and Robert C. Stanton. "High Glucose Inhibits Glucose-6-phosphate Dehydrogenase, Leading to Increased Oxidative Stress and ß-cell Apoptosis." The FASEB Journal (2010): 1497+. High Glucose Inhibits Glucose-6-phosphate Dehydrogenase, Leading to Increased Oxidative Stress and ß-cell Apoptosis. <www.fasebj.org, 9 June 2009. Web. 10 Apr. 2013. http://www.ncbi.nlm.nih.gov/pubmed/20032314>.

Index

Colophon

This cover and inside layout was done by Melody W. Baker, wife and helpmeet of Dale R. Baker. Melody also helped with much of the research and editing to insure the information contained in this book was as complete, accurate and up-to-date as possible.

About the Author

Dale R. Baker is a computer programmer by profession. After retirement, he started developing websites in his spare time. Because of health issues due to G6PD Deficiency and the lack of credible medical information, he developed g6pddeficiency.org to help bring others with this condition together to share their experiences. During the last six years, over 500,000 people have visited his website. He is a published writer and dedicated to helping people with this enzymopathy live a better life. His favorite hobby is cooking.

www.ingramcontent.com/pod-product-compliance
Lightning Source LLC
Chambersburg PA
CBHW070536290526
45790CB00002B/519